HEALING BEYOND THE DIAGNOSIS
Volume 1

19 HEALTH EXPERTS SIMPLIFY HOW YOU CAN SOLVE YOUR HEALTH PUZZLE

By Kylie Burton and Colleagues

Contributing to this book are:
Mike Rhees
Sarah Outlaw, MH
Jamie Pacini
Chantell Spohr, FNP-C
Dr. Kenna S. Ducey-Clark, DC
Dr. Mark R. Shane DC
Sandy Wesson BSN
Dr. Angela Rahm BCND
Sydney Torres, FDNP
Patty Jo Burress
Kristie Hess-Newton
Jessica Milner, MSHN
Tracy Chamber
Dina Rabo, DC
James E. Hicks, DC
Deniece Krebs, CHC
Jessica Watterud, LPCC
Renee Swasey

Copyright 2023 Kylie Burton
All Rights Reserved

ISBN: 979-8860590-54-0

Table of Contents

Healing Beyond the Diagnosis **Vol. 1** v

Chapter 1: We've Been Lied To
 By: Dr. Kylie Burton, DC, CFMP 1

Chapter 2: Getting to the True Root Cause
 By Sarah Outlaw, MH, MSACN 13

Chapter 3: Choosing Your Peace
 By Jamie Pacini 29

Chapter 4: What I Wish I Knew Before My Dad's Cancer Diagnosis
 By Chantell Spohr, FNP-C 37

Chapter 5: The Healing Path to Health and Reverse Aging
 By: Dr. Kenna S. Ducey-Clark, D.C., P.C. 45

Chapter 6: It's Not Your Thyroid
 By: Dr. Mark R. Shane, D.C. 71

Chapter 7: Healing the Body to Heal the Brain
 By: Sandy Wesson BSN, RN, FNTP, CGP 83

Chapter 8: Wellness to Weight Loss
 By: Dr. Angela Rahm B.C.N.D. 103

Chapter 9: Trial and Error Health
 By: Sydney Torres, FDNP 115

Chapter 10: Let's Make it Personal
            By: Patty Jo Burress 129

Chapter 11: From Wheelchair to Walking
            By: Kristie Hess-Newton 147

Chapter 12: The Relationship Between Gut and Hormones
            By: Jessica Milner, MSHN, FBWS 167

Chapter 13: Western and Eastern Medicine
            By: Tracy Chambers 175

Chapter 14: Case Study: Andrea, Age 52
            By: Dina Rabo, DC 181

Chapter 15: Four Quick Strategies to Improve Gut Function
            By: James E. Hicks, DC, CFMP 185

Chapter 16: The Code of YOU
            By: Deniece Krebs, CHC 197

Chapter 17: Depression & Anxiety and the Thyroid Connection
            By: Jessica Watterud, LPCC 231

Chapter 18: Your Health Puzzle
            By: Renee Swasey 239

Chapter 19: Microscopic Maestros
            By: Mike Rhees 249

Healing Beyond the Diagnosis
Vol. 1

Disclaimer: *This book shares personal experiences and provides education from Dr. Kylie and her colleagues. Interaction with this book does not constitute a doctor/ patient relationship and is not intended to diagnose, cure or treat any ailment. Where a condition is identified or a lab result is outside the normal range, the patient should seek appropriate conventional medical management and drug administration by a physician.*

CHAPTER 1:

We've Been Lied To

By: Dr. Kylie Burton, DC, CFMP

We've been lied to. We've been made to believe we should chase a diagnosis. We've been made to think that a diagnosis is an answer.

It's a lie.

All a diagnosis tells us is our symptoms fall underneath an umbrella term. If our symptoms don't fit a certain criteria, then we are told nothing is wrong with us or we are left hanging in the dark with no answers or relief.

Stop searching for a diagnosis. In fact, stop trying to treat your symptoms too. Stop asking google, "what causes *x, y, z*?" If there was a one-size-fits-all answer, you wouldn't get a trillion responses when you ask Google that one question.

Seeking a diagnosis has failed us. Treating symptoms has failed us.

What we really need to treat is the body as a whole. We all have incredible bodies, which, like I remind my six-year-old son almost daily when he gets an *owie*, "our body's are incredible at healing. You just have to give it the right tools and let it do what it was designed to do."

We've lost that knowledge: our body's are designed to heal. We've been inundated with tools of management. "If you have this, go tell your doctor you need this." Now it's not just the insurance telling doctors how to treat, it's commercials and Google too. Why can't we focus more on providing our body the tools it needs to heal rather than some concoction that helps us manage our symptoms? I don't care if it's a concoction of natural products or pharmaceuticals, it's still a concoction.

Look inside your supplement cupboard. How many are you taking? How much money are you spending on them? And why? Your best friend said this worked for her so you should try it too. Google says this product relieves your symptoms so you add it to the list. Your holistic practitioner makes suggestions too and those get added on.

Can I teach you a better way? I believe there is. Let me show you what can happen when you stop searching for a diagnosis. Let me show you what can happen when you stop managing your diagnosis.

Let me begin with Stephanie's story (name has been changed). It's one that many can resonate with. She's in her early sixties and can't seem to find help from anyone or anything. After finding my podcast, "Beyond the Diagnosis with Dr. Kylie," she emailed my team and explained a little of her journey:

"This has been the most frustrating process ever. I've even tried hormone therapy and that didn't do anything. All my blood work comes back normal and my doctors are thinking I'm crazy and just need an antidepressant. There's something wrong and I know it, but nobody will listen."

How many people have heard something similar? Is this you?

Other messages I've received or heard countless times from individuals are:

1- "I feel the doctors are just brushing me off. They don't know what to do so they dismiss the way I feel."

2- "Dr. Kylie, I am one of these people. Got sick about a year ago out of the blue when I felt the best in my life. Been to many doctors, had more blood drawn than I've ever had. Always normal I guess. Then some stuff showed up and still no answers. Rheumatologist just blew it off like it was nothing even though it concerned my GP. I have a lot of unexplained symptoms. It's really frustrating. I don't look sick but I am. I've become a shell of a man I was a year ago."

If this is you or similar to your story, you are in the right place. Just as Stephanie felt when she found me:

"I am excited and hopeful that we can get me straightened out. I prayed God would give me a sign on how to find out what is going on with me and I can't tell you how many times he slapped me in the face with your name, your podcasts, your posts, so let this process begin with His Blessing."

My process begins with two things:

1- a questionnaire so I know how people feel and
2- retrieving all the "normal" blood work they've received throughout the years.

Why? I have learned "normal" blood work has a GOLD MINE of answers if you know how to read it correctly. I read it correctly and even teach others how to read it correctly too. It saves people oodles of time and money. Not to mention I am like a kid on Christmas morning when I get a good set of labs. It makes my day.

Stephanie's labs were some good ones! Here's what I found in them:
- Blood Sugar Imbalances (which leads to hormone chaos)
- A need for hydrochloric acid in her stomach (a lack of which can lead to acid reflux)
- A struggling detox system as many kidney and liver markers were outside the functional ranges I prefer to see

- Adrenal fatigue (yes, I don't need a fancy test to determine this)
- Major signs of leaky gut, as all three markers in her labs were not in the functional range
- A need for more healthy fats
- Surprisingly, her vitamin D wasn't terrible but it could be better. I'm a huge fan of vitamin D levels being over 80—yes, you heard me right. (Nor do I care if they're over 100.)
- Gut and liver problems as indicated by her thyroid markers
- A possible need for more iron
- B vitamins were not being used efficiently
- And the big ones: bacterial and viral infections

The hormone lab tests she received were a very minor piece of the puzzle. As noted previously, she's tried hormone therapy and worked with a functional medicine specialist in hormones. No change in how she felt.

When I saw her questionnaire, I knew why. There's more to healing than fixing your hormones. The endocrine system is just one system. Your body is made up of multiple systems that all play together. We want them to play together nicely.

On the questionnaire I use, a 4 means the symptom is frequent and severe. Here are all the symptoms she listed at a 4:

- Chronic coughing
- Rapid or pounding heartbeat
- Chest pain
- Shortness of breath
- Diarrhea
- Constipation
- Bloated feeling
- Belching, passing gas
- Heartburn

- Craving certain foods
- Excessive weight
- Water retention
- Fatigue
- Mood swings
- Anxiety
- Depression
- Irritability

Notice how many symptoms are related to her GI (gastrointestinal) tract. Not one ounce of hormone therapy is going to fix that and the GI tract needs to be fixed first.

How do I fix it? Go back to her blood work. It tells me she's fighting a bacterial and viral infection. I know these bacterial infections can wreak havoc on guts and the viral infection causes major fatigue, anxiety and depression. But that's not all. Infections can wreak havoc anywhere the body is weak. This is just one piece of her healing journey, but it's a big one.

Going back and forth between how she feels and what her numbers tell me, I created a personalized six-month supplement plan for her. This plan is not intended to treat a diagnosis or a symptom. Its intent is to help her body heal. Its intent is to help each system, organ, tissue, gland, cell in the body function optimally. The body is one incredible machine with pieces that work together. Each piece needs to play its role and there's so much crossover that if you're just treating one system, you're getting things wrong.

Inside her six month plan, she knew from the very beginning every supplement she'd be taking, how much, when, and why. Because that's the way I roll. There's no guessing on my part. The blood work tells me what her body needs to heal. Your blood work can do the same—if you are reading it correctly.

If you're a practitioner reading this, you may be thinking, "what if the plan needs adjustment along the way?"

While this can happen, it rarely does. Numbers never lie and when you read blood work the way I do, I can be very confident in my treatment plans. In fact, Stephanie, like many others, are able to do this on their own with just a little support from me. I'm able to help more people this way.

Here's what she said after coming to the conclusion of her six-month plan, "gut is much better. I no longer take my medications and so feeling this good without them is awesome! I just have to watch out for BBQ and spaghetti sauce. They still give me heartburn but that's it. I'm so glad I did this and I'm hoping Dr. Kylie tells me what I need to do after this 6 month program to keep the gut problems far away. I like the way I feel—I don't want to go back."

Stephanie isn't the only person who has experienced healing from unknown symptoms. A diagnosis would not have served her. It probably isn't serving you well either.

Liz (name has been changed), also found me on my podcast, "Beyond the Diagnosis with Dr. Kylie." When she reached out, she had just experienced her first seizure. Being in her mid-20s, she knew this was not something she simply wanted to manage her entire life.

I've actually worked with a handful of seizure scenarios over the last year. I love to look at their blood work (like everyone else) and play detective to discover the trigger of these seizure episodes.

Since this was her first seizure, she had only one set of labs and it had been taken shortly after the episode, so in my opinion, prime time.

One marker really stood out to me: the Neutrophil count. It was 88%!!! I like to see it around 60% so this was quite high.

The blood work was taken while at the Emergency Room and gratefully, they gave it to her so she had it while at home, which we referenced. However, the ER didn't do anything about the blood work nor did they provide a report besides "it looks good."

Why? Because they don't know what to do about an elevated marker. If they were to show you a marker that was out of normal range (and probably way outside the functional range), you'd immediately ask, "what do we do about it?" If they don't know, why would they show you? Nor is it their fault. It's the education and training they receive. They're doing their best with the tools they have in their pocket. I've loaded my pocket with different tools. It's because of these tools that I can get different results. I want my colleagues to get different results too so I teach them my tools as well.

Anyways, back to the Neutrophil count. What does this mean? Bacterial infection. Without having any other background on her besides the one seizure episode, I asked if she had any gut complaints? That's when I learned there's a lot more to her health story than just the seizures.

Remember, I don't treat diagnoses. I don't treat symptoms. I help a body in an unhealthy state get healthy again and I believe everyone can heal. She's no different despite the symptom being a "scary one."

After reading her blood work, learning about her gut problems, and dialing in a treatment plan, the only way to find out if the neutrophil count has anything to do with the seizure episodes is to treat. So we did.

Ninety days later, here's what she had to say, "my gut was a mess! So bad I ended up in the ER a couple of times. They'd always send me home without any answers or relief. My stomach would hurt every time I ate, as it wouldn't digest anything. After trying a million supplements, I did Dr. Kylie's program. It has changed the way my gut functions. I took a complete 180 in just 90 days and now I feel AMAZING!"

The seizures are still a work in progress but every time an episode comes around, if given the chance, I correlate it to her blood work. Without a doubt, the neutrophil count was elevated again. I know one big key to her staying healthy with very little episodes, if any, is to keep that neutrophil count down around 60 and we do that with some supplements.

I would have never known any of this if I didn't read the blood work she kept getting told was normal. Your blood work is loaded with golden nuggets too if you have the right person reading it.

Now that I've convinced you a diagnosis is not an answer nor a life sentence, let me also convince you to stop owning your diagnosis like it's something you can't live without.

Be careful how you talk about it. Saying "I have Hashimoto's" gives up your power to heal and turns it over to your disease. Be careful how you talk about your body's health struggle. Are you giving the struggle more power or are you giving the power to your body to heal?

Let me give you an example.

I received a message from an individual on my Facebook one day. It was a voice memo and I'm always hesitant to open those. This one I knew was going to be loaded.

It was from a young mom who fought severe depression with every child she's had. This was after baby number two but pregnancy number three. We've had conversations before so I knew I needed to get my head in the right space for this one. So I did and I pressed play on the message.

Without typing it up word for word, she told me about her new health concerns and what had led her to be in this state. Her voice was shaky as she fought back tears while explaining this to me:

"My mind is playing games with me. I need it fixed and I need it fixed like yesterday. I see an [alternative practitioner] this week as a friend recommended them but I was hoping to get your advice first."

I'm always happy to help. However, we had a few major mind blocks we needed to heal before any physical healing would take place and people don't like to hear this. Oftentimes, we want to skip this part and just want to heal physically with some form of treatment.

I jumped on the phone with her. On rare occasions I do this. She was in a very desperate situation—possibly leading to hospitalization for her depression if we didn't do something fast.

Now, I know what you're thinking. What supplement did I recommend to her? What can I give to her that'll kick her out of this state and kick it fast?

Spoiler alert: nothing.

No supplement on this earth (or pharmaceutical) would be able to fix the state she was in.

Why? She had given all her power to her illness and her recent postpartum diagnosis. I could hear it in the story she told me over and over again. In fact, I got to a point where I couldn't listen to it anymore. The story she told was keeping her in this state of depression as she allowed it to consume her and to take all power from her.

After providing her with some other options of healing, which she declined because they weren't going to fix her overnight (if you know of something that does, they're a billionaire by now), I guided her to attend this appointment she had scheduled and to let me know what they said.

I was very familiar with the mechanism and treatment of this alternative practitioner but as always, people need to experience it for themselves.

After receiving an energetic scan, her results came up with red in nearly every column - every part of her body was not doing well. According to this scan, there were plenty of reasons why she felt the way she did.

Using the scan, the practitioner placed her on a few homeopathics and sent her on her way, advising her to come back in a month and they'd make alterations to the supplement regimen. So she followed the advice, went home, and started the regimen.

She contacted me shortly after arriving back home as I told her I wanted to know what they said and what the plan was.

Now, in the alternative health world, we all have different modalities, specialties, and ways we do business. I prefer to tell my patients the entire plan from the get-go. They know everything we will be doing up front, down to the supplement they're taking each month (when, what, how much, and why) throughout the entire healing journey. I use their regular blood work to help me create this toolkit their body needs to heal; just as you've seen in the last two examples.

As I learned of this "lack of plan," I wasn't impressed. But again, to each their own. Let me also reiterate that no supplement or pharmaceutical was going to help in this scenario. She had some deep inner work to do and at this point, unwilling to even try it.

Unfortunately, my prediction was right. She gave the story and the diagnosis so much power, telling everyone who would listen about it. Her husband ended up taking her into the hospital a few days after meeting with this practitioner. Gratefully the hospital helped her create a plan and get on some medication to help her get through these rough times.

To avoid rough times ahead, she'll be starting my new "90-day Whole Body Healing Program" soon. I'm excited for her as it's all encompassing and does exactly what it says it does: heals the whole body.

Will I be treating her postpartum depression diagnosis? No.

Will I be treating her as a whole person, helping her go from unhealthy to healthy? Yes.

To get the best results, you, like her, will need more than supplements, pharmaceuticals, a fancy dietary regimen, and whatever you can do physically. She needs to dig down deep and heal her inner self. To start, she'll learn the power of story and how changing the way she tells her story will change the power she's giving to her diagnosis.

She FOUGHT postpartum depression but now she's healing. She KNOWS her body can heal.

I believe you can heal. You need to believe it too.

So stop chasing that diagnosis.

Stop trying to treat or manage symptoms.

Stop telling yourself (and everyone else) you have this diagnosis or illness. Don't give it any power over you.

Your body can heal. Believe it. Like my six-year-old son, I'm here to tell you it can heal and it's very good at healing.

Dive inside each chapter of this book and learn what those tools can be to truly heal. Each chapter is written by a colleague of mine who has become a "Functional Blood Work Specialist" and I know you'll be in safe hands with any of them.

Dr. Kylie

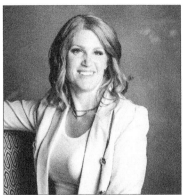

Dr. Kylie Burton, DC, CFMP, is an international best-seller with her book *Why are My Labs Normal?* She specializes in functional medicine helping thousands of individuals with seemingly impossible health struggles, find answers, healing, and hope, even if they've been told their blood work is normal.

As the founder of the "Functional Blood Work Specialist" program for practitioners, she helps colleagues level up their patient results and build a business they love using her techniques in her programs.

Dr. Kylie hosts the top-rated podcast Beyond the Diagnosis with Dr. Kylie. Dr. Kylie has been featured on seven international radio shows. On TV, she has been a guest on Good Morning Utah and FOX26Houston, and The List (national TV).

Besides running a successful business, Kylie keeps herself plenty busy as a wife and mother of three young children. She loves spending time outdoors and has many years of playing and coaching volleyball under her belt.

→ For those without medical background—you can be the best person to read your own labs, go here and she'll teach you: bloodworkspecialist.com/labs

→ If you are a practitioner and want to become a certified Functional Blood Work Specialist like the authors in this book, join the next 90-day program here: drkylieburton.com/90

CHAPTER 2:

Getting to the True Root Cause

By Sarah Outlaw, MH, MSACN

You can't pour from an empty cup. You just can't. Trust me, I tried.

Let's have a conversation. Motherhood demands tremendous energy. So does fulfilling roles as a wife or partner, a businesswoman, and all the other responsibilities you juggle. Falling ill is simply not an option. Nor is accepting being told that nothing is wrong when deep down, you sense otherwise. It's crucial to grasp the reins of your health. You must discover the true root cause of whatever is impeding your journey towards living your most fulfilling life. This is non-negotiable.

You are not your diagnosis! Or, your lack of one.

My story may echo yours. It's a narrative that could strike a chord with many of you as you delve into its details.

Once upon a time, I was not a practitioner; instead, I was that weary mother, relentlessly attempting to pour from an empty cup, for years. Unbeknownst to me, I grappled with a chronic illness, unaware of its existence. All I knew was an overwhelming fatigue and exhaustion. It wasn't until I found healing and experienced the true wellness that I realized how profoundly I had needlessly suffered.

Let's rewind a few years when I was a little girl. I had stomach issues all of the time. I grew up in an Italian family and on Sundays we always had spaghetti. I would feel so sick after eating and I would have to go upstairs and lay down on my stomach. In college this continued and got worse. I had such horrible stomach issues that I would not go to the bathroom for weeks.

Literally weeks. I had so much gas and bloating and constipation that I was in agony all of the time, but I was too embarrassed to tell anyone about it. It became my normal.

When I was twenty-years-old, I moved to Germany with my new husband as an army wife. I took a job at a veterinary treatment facility on base and for that job, I was required to get some vaccines. Little did I know that those vaccines would send my health into a crazy tailspin. You see, when I was seven years old I was bitten by a tick. What I did not realize was that at that time I contracted a tick borne illness that lay dormant in my system just waiting for the right moment to cause me serious problems. When I got those vaccines, that tick borne illness activated and from that point on I was sick. Really sick. I gained weight. I was constantly tired. I had horrible migraines. I could barely get up. I had trouble putting sentences together and I would stutter when I was tired. I had extreme brain fog.

I went to the doctor on base and told him my symptoms. He did no testing at all. He simply looked at me and said that I was depressed and that I should just take an antidepressant and I would be fine. I told him no, I am not depressed. I'm having the time of my life. I just got married. I am living in a beautiful country. I have a wonderful job, and I'm having fun traveling and doing amazing things. Things that I would love to be able to do more of but I am too tired and weak to do them. He insisted that I was just depressed and that I should just take this antidepressant and I would be fine. Even at twenty-years-old, I knew better. I walked out of that office very discouraged, but determined to find out what was wrong with me. I didn't know what was wrong with me, and I had no resources at that time to find out.

I got pregnant with my oldest daughter and five weeks after she was born we moved back to the United States. I took her to the pediatrician for a well visit where I was informed that she was behind on her vaccines. I did not know any better or what I know now so I allowed them to give her five vaccines, some of which were combo vaccines. She had a reaction. I did not realize how that reaction would carry over into her life later on with gut and metabolic issues.

A little over a year after having her I had a miscarriage. Then I got pregnant with my son shortly after. After having him I had another miscarriage and then I had another baby a couple of years later. This continued. All in all, I have had five miscarriages. Every time I would have a baby my health would crash.

I began to look for someone who could help me that was more holistic minded. I did not want a repeat of the on-base physician from a few years before. I had started studying holistic health and nutrition and had become a health coach so I was super interested in knowing how to help myself and also to be the primary caregiver for my children.

I had learned about muscle testing and how it could possibly help me. I started with a muscle testing practitioner in California. I immediately started seeing some progress on some symptoms that I was having including the extreme fatigue, cystic acne from ear to ear and I felt like I was gaining some ground physically and mentally. We then had to move back to New Jersey again and there wasn't anyone there that I could find who did this muscle testing technique. So I was on my own again.

I was asked by my chiropractor at that time to come on board with him to be a nutrition coach there. I decided to go back to school and get my master's degree in clinical nutrition, an equivalent to a master's degree in herbal medicine, and also go to school to learn muscle testing because I knew how much that had helped me previously. I wanted to be able to help people just as I had been helped.

While in muscle testing school I finally got answers. I had Lyme disease. I had Epstein Barr. I had parasites, I had hypothyroidism. I had heavy metal toxicity from aluminum and mercury. I had all of these things going on in my body that were affecting my ability to be a mother the way I was meant to be, the wife I wanted to be, the vibrant life I was meant to live. Once I found answers, I knew that I had to do this for the rest of my life.

All of those years trying to pour from an empty cup, I was finally able to start filling it. I was able to get the help I needed, the proper nutrition, the proper herbs and finally was able to be me again. What happens many times in the conventional health world is that doctors dismiss what patients say. They brushed it off. It's no big deal. Bloodwork lies. My labs told me I was fine. My labs never told doctors anything other than my thyroid was a little off. It didn't show that my adrenals were tired. It didn't show that my mitochondria was tired. It didn't show that I had Lyme. It didn't show enough for them to be alarmed. So I had to suffer for years. This is not okay. For me. For anyone.

Before finding the natural health world, I was going down a path of conventional health. I used tons of Lysol in my house thinking that if I didn't keep everything clean that my kids would get sick. I vaccinated for everything until a friend of mine introduced me to the real truth that I could possibly be harming my children. I never put two and two together that the vaccines that I got when I was twenty could have contributed to my poor health. I did not know that until very much later in life. So from age twenty to age thirty-five, I lived in the dark when it came to my own health. It wasn't until I started to get the help that I needed that I understood that what I had done with those vaccines at twenty activated something in my body that caused a chain reaction that actually negatively affected my eldest daughter in utero. I got pregnant with her less than a year from getting those vaccines and actually passed on some of that heavy metal toxicity to her. That toxicity contributed to her having those vaccine reactions when she was just a couple months Old.

People always say that when you know better, you do better. And this is the case with me. I did not know that putting those vaccines into my body would destroy my health. I thought I was helping my health. I thought that vaccinating my children was the right thing to do because I was told if I didn't, I would get CPS called on me. I was told that I was endangering my children If I did not vaccinate them. It wasn't until I did my own research that I realized the damage that I had done to myself and possibly my children. I barely remember age twenty to thirty-five. That's how damaged my cells were. That's how tired and fatigued my body was, trying to figure out what to do with all this autoimmunity.

So how does my story benefit *you*? Well, it benefits you because if you're reading this, and you are tired and exhausted and feel like you can't fill from an empty cup like I was, then I have help and hope for you. I found the answers when no one else could. Now I have helped thousands of people find answers to their health concerns and questions. Over the last ten years I have made it my mission to educate parents on how to take care of themselves and their children naturally, and how to get to the root cause of their health issues.

What saved me? What allowed me to get my health back? Ultimately, Muscle Testing.

I practice an advanced form of muscle testing that gets to the root cause of common symptoms. Some of the things we commonly help to resolve in my practices are asthma, eczema, allergies, ADD, ADHD, psoriasis. digestive issues, autoimmune issues, skin issues, chronic illness, Lyme, Epstein Barr, cytomegalovirus, chronic fatigue and so much more. Everything you have going on that would be considered a symptom or a diagnosis has an underlying root cause. Once you identify what that cause is, you are then finally able to heal.

The 7 most common root causes:

1. Underlying immune system issues/ Food sensitivities

First let's talk about food sensitivities. Just cutting out food is not the answer. Now, here me out. Most people go about food sensitivities the wrong way. They think that just by eliminating foods, they will completely heal what's going on symptom-wise. Food sensitivities are not actually the root cause. They are another symptom but they are worth looking at because that is usually what people will notice when they have something going on in their bodies. A food sensitivity can be causing a stomach ache. It can cause skin rashes. It can cause ear aches. It can cause all sorts of different reactions in the body. These are your body's way of saying hey, there's something going on. I need to fix it. For me, I was sensitive to every food except a few meats and some vegetables. Fruit would make me fall asleep, and rice would cause my legs to not be able to move. Wheat and sugar? Sick for days with migraines.

Here, we are talking about a parasitic imbalance, or a virus, bacteria, fungus or something that is going on underneath that's causing the body to have an immune system reaction to the food that you're eating. Most food sensitivities are not true allergies. They are usually an inflammatory response, or a sensitivity. What we commonly find is that if we fix the immune system and the gut, whatever the food sensitivities are, they will go away in about 90 to 120 days, by eliminating them temporarily and fixing the root cause.

These things are also root causes to many other biological processes in the body that contribute to symptoms. Once we identify those, we can help the immune system become supported and help the gut and those issues also go away. Even the tough stuff! Even Lyme, Epstein Barr, and mold illness.

2. Heavy metal and chemical toxicity

Heavy Metal and chemical toxicity very often causes a viral type reaction in the body. Viruses are actually exosomes, meaning that they are an immune system reaction activated by a toxin. Let's take glyphosate otherwise known as roundup as an example. I have many patients in my practices that have displayed virus-like symptoms after being exposed to glyphosate on a baseball field or at a park or playing on a farm. They didn't actually have a virus. They had a toxicity that was causing a virus-like reaction. This may not be a commonly known reaction to a chemical, but it is something that we are seeing every day. Heavy metals also cause huge issues. Most of the heavy metals that I find in patients come from either childhood or current vaccines. They come from the workplace that they are in every day. They come from mercury amalgam fillings in their mouths. They come from their cleaning products or their personal care products, etc. Muscle testing helps us to actually identify what these are. Then we can confidently figure out what the sources are to help people not be continually exposed while we're detoxing their bodies.

3. Emotions

Emotional distress causes stress in the body that can manifest physically. We do an emotional technique in my practice called

"Body Code," which helps us to untangle these emotional baggage type situations so the body can release things that are no longer serving them and begin to heal.

4. Mold

I mentioned this earlier. I like to actually put mold into a category by itself because it's so insidious. Mold enters the body usually from the environment. It can cause a lot of problems health-wise, including toxicity, neurological issues, breathing issues, skin issues. The really cool thing about the testing I do is that I can find out very easily if someone ate it in, breathed it in, or if it's chronic or acute exposure. There's also functional lab testing that can go along with muscle testing to see if someone has mold in their system.

5. Scars

These are another thing that we look for because they cause nerve interference. About 90% of the nerve fibers that talk to the autonomic nervous system (the system that runs the body) are located on the surface of the skin. When you cut through, pierce or tattoo the skin, you cut through those nerve fibers. This causes problems in how the body heals. Think of it like a letter that never gets to its intended recipient or an email that bounces. Information about your environment gets stuck in the scar like energy getting stuck in a capacitor and never gets to where it needs to go. This can contribute to the body not being able to heal.

6. The Autonomic Nervous System

Everything we do is very much autonomic nervous system based. The autonomic nervous system is a system that runs the body. It does all of the things that you don't have to think about doing everyday like making your eyes blink, your heart beat, or your lungs breathe. You have two main parts to your autonomic nervous system that need to work together to run your body.

You have the sympathetic part of the nervous system, which is like your body's gas pedal. It's moving, talking, heart rate, blood pressure, stress response…all the active things your body does. You also have the parasympathetic part of your nervous system. This is more of your body's brake pedal so think of it in more of a passive way. Think of it like resting, digesting and healing.

They each have different jobs. They have to work together to run the body well and they run on the nutrition your body brings in as their fuel. So if your nutrition is either not right for you, you're not absorbing or assimilating or digesting what you're eating very well, or if there is a toxicity in your body blocking your nutrition, the parasympathetic and sympathetic parts of the nervous system will not work well together. Your organs will get very unhappy, they will begin to dysfunction and symptoms will appear. Once you have a symptom, there's been something going on for a while that the body has been trying to fix on its own but can't so it sends up those symptoms like a little red flag saying, hey, I need some help here. That's where I come in. My job is to get to the root cause of someone's symptoms, find out what's going on at that deeper level and help the body fix it.

7. Medications

Pharmaceuticals bypass the body's autonomic nervous system and force the body to make a change. Nutrition nourishes the autonomic nervous system and allows the body to fix itself by giving it the tools that it needs. Conventional medicine will see a symptom as something to be squashed or covered up. Think of your car's engine light. When your engine light is on, if you just put a sticky note over that check engine light what happens? The check engine light is still on and whatever is causing that check engine light to come on is still a problem. You're just covering it up. If you treat a symptom with medication without finding the root cause, you are simply putting a sticky note or a bandaid over that symptom and what's going on underneath that symptom is still happening. If you ignore your check engine light in your car, your engine will eventually blow up. If you ignore the symptoms in your body, your health will continue to decline. We don't want that. We want to help get to the root cause of anything that's happening in the body, so we can take care of it and live a healthy life.

So how do we do this? How do we combine muscle testing and functional labs in our practice to give someone the best results?

Well, let's talk about muscle testing first. What is muscle testing? Muscle testing is a non-invasive way of getting to the root cause of symptoms by identifying the real problems. We identify food sensitivities, immune system challenges, heavy metal toxicity, chemical toxicity, scars, mold and emotions. Those are the main seven things that we address. Once we find those things. We look for the remedies for those things. Those remedies are going to be nutritional supplements, herbs, products made from with carbon technology, dietary changes, nutrition, etc.

To understand muscle testing, think of someone who has hypothermia. When they come out of the cold water, their fingers and toes and arms and legs are numb because all of the energy, blood flow and circulation will leave what you can live without, your fingers and toes, and move towards what you can't live without for long, like your heart, your liver and your lungs. So, if I were standing in front of you, I'm not under any stress. If you walk over to me and you push on my arm I could easily resist you just like if I pushed on your arm, you could easily resist me.

If there's something going on with an organ like my heart, for example, and you walk over to me and you push on my heart and my arm at the same time, my arm would actually collapse because the energy, blood flow and circulation would leave my hand and move towards my heart to protect it.

Just like if I touched a hot stove. I don't have to think about my hand sitting there burning while it burns. I would move my hand out the way really fast because it's hot. That is actually part of your autonomic nervous system's job to protect your body from getting hurt more than it needs to. So we use that protection mechanism to test for stress in your entire system. I use your arm as your strength indicator. I push on each organ in the body. If the arm stays strong, there's no stress. If the arm goes weak, there's some kind of stress I have to find. I identify the organs and areas that come up as stressed, find the one that's the most stressed, and then I have to find out why. In person testing will use testing vials which have liquid representations of different possibilities.

Everything I do is biochemistry and physics. The physics portion of the testing is looking for the actual issue with the vials. Instead of doing an allergist version of a scratch test, patch tests or even blood testing initially, I use the non-invasive muscle testing to figure out what someone has going on. So with the vials I test with I look for the food sensitivities, I check for bacteria, viruses, fungus, yeast, molds, parasites.

The precision of my testing is pretty incredible. Once I pinpoint what someone has going on at the root cause of their health, I know exactly the right protocol for them to go on. I know the exact right foods for them to be eating. Once I put together an individualized protocol, I will have labs drawn and we go over those results together in the functional ranges to see just what the blood is really doing.

This is a key component to what I do, educating patients on what those numbers really mean in relationship to each other and as a whole. A holistic approach to Health. Muscle testing and labs. It's a beautiful combination! And it gets incredible results.

How Can Muscle Testing Be Done Virtually?

Einstein said, "Future medicine will be the medicine of frequencies." Using this concept, muscle testing can also be done virtually. Since it's frequency based and everything in life has a frequency, I can actually test someone from across the room, across the country, or across the world. We call it distance testing. Think of Einstein's theory of E=MC2. There is no "D" (Distance) in the equation of energy. Why? Energy is everywhere. It just goes where it wants. Through computers, cell phone towers, etc. it can go anywhere. So utilizing the same frequencies, I can test someone no matter where they are.

For years, I struggled to pour from an empty cup, but finally, I realized that I needed to take care of myself first. I learned the importance of getting to the true root cause of my health issues and addressing them directly. This journey taught me that healing is a holistic process that encompasses not only physical health but also mental, emotional, and spiritual well-being.

What if I hadn't taken matters into my own hands? What if I hadn't looked for the answers to solve my own health issues? Where would my life be now? I honestly don't know if I would be here because my health was declining with chronic issues left unchecked. I know for sure that my quality of life would have continued to go downhill, I would never have been able to open a successful practice and then another one, and then another one. I would never have been able to travel around the country teaching what I do to thousands of other practitioners. I would never have been able to travel back-and-forth every other week to my Des Moines clinic for almost three years. I would never have been able to thrive with that type of busy lifestyle.

I work with women who, like me, have struggled with chronic health issues and are searching for answers. I work with their children, their spouses, their pets. Together, we dig deep into their health history, perform comprehensive lab tests, and utilize techniques such as muscle testing to identify underlying imbalances and root causes.

What about you? Where is your health right now? What if you don't do anything about your health? Where do you see yourself in five years? Ten years? What does your quality of life look like when you are sixty-five, seventy-five, eighty-five? Are you the elderly person still driving and going to social functions in their 80's, or are you the elderly person in a nursing home? The choices you make now determine that for you.

One of the most common challenges I encounter with my clients is the misdiagnosis or dismissal of their symptoms by conventional medical practitioners. Many of them have been told that nothing is wrong or that their symptoms are merely a result of stress or aging. But deep down, they know that something is off. They can't accept the idea of feeling exhausted, in pain, or mentally foggy as their new normal. Getting to the true root cause requires a comprehensive approach. It involves looking beyond the surface-level symptoms and delving into a person's lifestyle, diet, environmental exposures, emotional well-being, and genetic predispositions. It means considering the interconnectedness of various body systems and how imbalances in one area can affect others. Through personalized protocols that include targeted nutrition, lifestyle modifications, stress management techniques, and natural therapies, I help my clients address the underlying imbalances and support their body's innate healing abilities. We work together as a team, empowering them to take control of their health and make informed decisions about their well-being.

I believe that every individual deserves to live a life of vitality and fulfillment. It's not about just surviving or managing symptoms; it's about thriving and truly living. By getting to the true root cause of health issues, we can unlock the potential for transformation and allow individuals to reclaim their vitality and live their best lives.

So, if you find yourself pouring from an empty cup, feeling like something is off, or being dismissed by the medical system, know that there is hope. Seek out practitioners who are willing to listen, explore, and dig deep to find the true root cause of your health concerns. Remember, you deserve to live a life of vibrant health, and with the right support and guidance, you can achieve it.

If my story of health and healing and how I went from barely surviving to thriving inspires you to take control of your own health, I invite you to work with me. My story can be your story too. Let me help you get to the true root cause for you. Natural Health Improvement Centers offer in-person and virtual consultations.

Visit www.nhiccenters.com to book an appointment for an initial consultation and testing that can be the first step in changing your health and your life today.

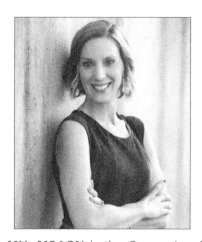

Sarah Outlaw, MH, MSACN is the Owner, Lead Practitioner & Director of Natural Health Improvement Center of Des Moines and South Carolina, and owner of Natural Health Improvement Center of South Jersey. She is a Functional, Clinical Herbalist and Nutritionist, holds a Master's Degree in Applied Clinical Nutrition from Northeast College of Health Sciences (formerly New York Chiropractic College), and is now pursuing her clinical doctorate. She has earned professional certificates as a Health Coach, Clinical, Master Herbalist, and Advanced Nutrition Response Testing® Practitioner. She is a Certified Emotion Code and Body Code Practitioner, Quantum Nutrition Testing Practitioner, and Advanced Cellcore Muscle Testing Practitioner. In addition to her busy, thriving Iowa in-person muscle testing and functional nutrition practice and two other practices in Mount Pleasant, South Carolina, and Cherry Hill, NJ. Sarah also has a virtual practice where she sees patients all over the world. Practitioner and patient education is a passion of hers so she also helps train and mentor fellow practitioners and teaches on a variety of topics to both practitioners and patients, including teaching muscle testing all over the country.

CHAPTER 3:

Choosing Your Peace

By Jamie Pacini

How to listen and understand your body, when the world is telling you there is nothing wrong

"Get up Jamie! Put your feet on the floor and get up!" It had been years of waking up day after day to this thought plaguing my mind, trying to convince myself and push past the emotional, mental, spiritual, and physical exhaustion I felt each morning … because … well … nothing was wrong... at least that is what I had been told visit after visit, year after year.

"Mom, are you okay?"

I opened my eyes just enough to see one of my littles standing next to my bed and I pulled them in to cuddle while the battling conversation to get up continued in my head. My brain was done fighting with my aching body.

I dozed off with my little one in my arms; I slept more than I was awake and I had accepted that this was my life.

After what seemed like forever, my little one moved. I gently kissed them, motivation enough for me to finally get up.

As I walked out into the hallway, wondering how I was going to make it through another day, I overheard two of my other kids talking at the bottom of the stairs:

"You know what I wish?"

"What?"

"That mom was more like ___," and named one of my friends "because she would play with us again."

Tears filled my eyes as the innocence spoken to the reality of what my life had become hit home and changed the trajectory of my life forever.

In each moment we are presented with choices. Easy choices. Hard choices. Choices we subconsciously do without thinking. Choices we say no to.

And that day, at that moment, I had a choice…

Now, I could sit here and explain the choice I made with all the steps associated with it, and though much would be helpful, in one chapter it would be way too much information. Not to mention the diversity of each of us, and being the unique individuals we are, it wouldn't allow you the proper tools to understand what YOU need and what YOUR body is saying.

I know … I know … food and the way we eat is important and we all need specific nutrients! Yes, finding what movement works for our unique body is key in so many aspects of healing. I know, and I love working with my clients on finding these avenues of support. But there is something that comes before any of that, something that if mastered will allow for the dreaded self sabotage to stay at bay, and instead of being another one of the 98% of people that fail to achieve optimal health, will set the stage for a solid foundation and put you in the 2% that find sustainable steps to truly living life.

… in that moment I could have chosen to continue to follow the motions, continue convincing myself that "nothing was wrong, it was all in my head" and exist through life, but that day I chose differently. That day I chose to believe that the life I wanted was possible, worth fighting for, that my body was trying to talk to me, and the tools to listen and understand were out there.

At that moment, no other doctors could tell me nothing was wrong, because I knew something was. In that moment I was filled with peace that my body, intricately designed, had the power and ability to heal itself, but I had to find the tools to tap into that. At that moment, no one else could tell me I was crazy or that I was a bad mom. And the only people I was willing to listen to were God and myself!

Our brain holds a lot of power and unless we believe we can heal and are ready to fight for ourselves like we would fight for those we love, then no process or plan I provide to you today will fully work.

So how did I go from following the motions to taking action? Let's start with a few basics you can start today to change the trajectory of your life, a few simple things that will move you towards living the life you want and seeing the results of believing it's possible!

Step One: Breathe ... just breathe!

Okay, okay, I know, you already know how to breathe. I get it, but hear me out, and stay away from the mindset of "I already know this", because even me, someone who has gone from unhealthy to healthy and someone who teaches and lives it, still needs the reminders and clarity at times to get back to the basics so I don't get complacent or fly off the rails.

To choose peace within ourselves to live life, the first thing we need to learn is breathing, but not just any form of breathing, mindful and conscious breathing!

When I was diagnosed with Lupus, my doctor told me that one of the leading causes of death in Lupus patience was stress and that I needed to find ways to reduce it. When my mom heard my diagnosis, she counseled me with the exact same advice, having had a friend pass from it.

Internal and external stress cause our sympathetic nervous system, or our flight, fight, or freeze response to be activated, telling our systems that something is wrong.

The crazy part about this system is that it doesn't matter if you are overwhelmed and stressed, being yelled at by someone, or getting chased by a bear ... the response is the same. Learning to turn this response off when the bear isn't there, will drastically help in reducing both external and internal stress; and we can do that through breathing.

Let's think about this for a second. What happens when panic, anxiety, fear, stress or anger kick in? The heart starts to beat faster, breathing shallows, logical thinking often shuts off and emotion thinking kicks in. And what does this have to do with healing our body? Everything! Because when our fight or flight response (sympathetic nervous system) is activated and we stay in that space, our rest and digest capabilities (or the parasympathetic nervous system) is shut off and our bodies are prevented from absorbing and digesting the needed nutrients from our food into our system. Not only that, but restful sleeping also becomes more difficult.

I know it sounds too good to be true, and way too simple, but breathing really is one of the keys to relaxation and stress release, which leads to a decrease in internal stress and inflammation.

Don't believe me, try it. I invite you to pause for a second right here, mark this page, and try it before moving on. Take a deep and slow breath in, hold it for a few seconds, and then slowly release the air until your lungs are empty, and then repeat the cycle of inhaling, holding your breath, and exhaling until you feel an internal shift (usually about ten mindful and slow breaths).

Or better yet, go out into nature, lay on the earth and ground yourself (putting your hands or bare feet on the ground and connect skin to skin to the earth) and breathe slowly and consciously for 10-15 minutes and notice what that does for you.

Step Two: Be realistic to what CAN and what CANNOT be controlled in our lives.

Reality is that most circumstances are outside of our control and we have no real say on what other people think or say about us. Yet how often do we take to heart the words or actions of others, and believe them?

Imagine a young child coming to you, scared and shaking from nightmares or self doubt because they have been bullied or in abusive situations. What would you do? For real, don't read any more until you really think about this question. What would you do?

I know for me, I would bend down, comfort the child, and let them know they are not alone and they are safe with me. And I would probably tell them not to listen to those other people because what they are saying isn't true.

So here is a question, why don't we do that with ourselves? Why don't we comfort and care for our own inner child that wants to feel safe? We were all once children, and that child is still a part of us, yet we so often listen to and accept what others say about us as truth, which shuts us down, makes us doubt or question ourselves, makes us think we are crazy, or convinces us how we should be feeling or handling our situation ... why?

My advice ... STOP IT! Honestly ... please stop it! Stop listening to them! They are not you! They have no idea the circumstances you are facing, the ups and downs, the pain and emotions that circulate through you. Trust me, you are NOT crazy! Your body is communicating with you, and once you can calm down your system enough to allow for clear thinking through breathing, you have to be willing to hear what YOUR BODY is saying and tune out everyone else's opinions!

Every time something is said that makes you feel less than, crazy, etc. I want you to do some conscious breathing and then, tell yourself, "I believe you." And mean it! It might be easy to believe or it might take time to wholeheartedly believe and that's ok. Neither is wrong, just honor yourself wherever you are right now.

Step Three: Understand your pain or illness is NOT you!

The last step in getting to a point of believing that healing is possible and being able to move forward to becoming that best version of you, is to understand that your pain or illness is not you!! Once upon a time you lived without pain, you didn't have the struggles you have today and that is because they are not who you are.

In those moments where the pain is too much, your exhaustion takes over, or you are struggling to be "normal", please remember that your system is struggling, but a struggling system does not mean that your soul, light, gifts, and talents all of a sudden disappear.

When I stood in the hallway all those years ago and heard my kids wish that I could be the mom that once played with them again, I paused. I took deep breaths. I decided I wasn't going to listen to the countless people who didn't believe me any more and I was going to listen to my body in figuring out what it needed. And in that moment I realized that no diagnosis would change my symptoms or where I was with everything going on. My body hurt. My brain was tired. And a diagnosis was just a name. So if there was no name, fine, there was still something wrong and I was going to figure out the "what" and the answer.

At that moment I began a journey of healing I never imagined possible. I found what foods added or took away my energy because I believed my body knew. I realized that movement looked different for everyone and found what worked for me. I came to understand the natural world and all the elements that heal and sustain. I learned the power in our body's makeup through Epigenetics and being able to read and assess blood work.

I went back to school because I wanted to become the mom my kids wanted and needed and not only because they wanted it, but because I WANTED it. Even if nothing else came from school, if I could learn the skills and tools to find healing in myself, that was enough.

Yet through the course of my learnings, I realized that what I was gaining couldn't be kept in, it was selfish, because if I would have known then, what I know now, I would have been able to live so much more of my life.

Don't take me wrong, I don't regret the time I took to get here because in that time I learned, grew, and became who I am today, but if I can help anyone … YOU … skip the steps of frustration, I will!

So where am I now? I am off medications for my Lupus and Rheumatoid Arthritis, my labs look amazing, and I love hiking and taking adventures with my kids. I am alive, living a full and meaningful life!

To all those who have lost hope, who believe they are stuck, or that life is just a stagnant place of pain and hurt, I would invite you to implement the three steps above into your life for 30 days and see what happens! By taking one simple step for change at a time, healing begins to happen. That's how we choose our own place of peace to reside in, enjoy the journey, and love each moment without the chaos swirling through us.

You are not alone! I was once there. You've got this … and I am here to help.

Feel free to tune into my podcast "Choosing Your Peace" on Spotify or Apple to hear more steps to achieving optimal health.

And for questions, please reach out and email me at: simplybeautifulwithjmi@gmail.com

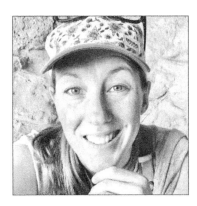

Jamie Michelle Pacini is a busy mom of four, loves her family, and loves her relationship with her Heavenly Parents and Savior Jesus Christ.

She loves the natural world, and takes every opportunity she can to spend time there! Whether gardening, hiking, camping, playing in streams & waterfalls, or just being, Jamie finds healing through Mother Nature. She also enjoys writing music and stories, singing, playing the piano, swimming, learning languages, and a good party.

Jamie personally understands the effects of sexual abuse, mental health struggles, and autoimmune disorders. Utilizing her education and personal knowledge & experience, she specializes in nature based healing that provides the tools, resources, and skills needed to guide women through different areas of healing.

She educates women on how to take control of their lives, understand what their unique bodies need, and helps rewire any blocks to positive beliefs that will support them in achieving success in life. By diving into nutrition, the brain/gut connection, and the benefits of the natural world to realign mind and body, her clients are able to create the life they want with a harmonious flow of joy and peace amongst the unexpected circumstances that show up!

Circumstances might be outside of our control, but choices are ours.

CHAPTER 4:

What I Wish I Knew Before My Dad's Cancer Diagnosis

By Chantell Spohr, FNP-C

When I first signed up to take nursing classes, I didn't know what to expect, I just knew I wanted to help people. Now, as a Family Nurse Practitioner, I had to go outside of my comfort zone to learn other avenues of care so I can actually help people and give them answers instead of band-aids. Now, don't get me wrong, medicine has its purpose, and it is not wrong, it just was not what I was looking for. Providers are just not taught what you are learning in this book. It is a whole different division in helping people restore their health. One in which I personally am grateful for.

A little over a year ago, in May 2022, I asked my father to complete a heart smart CT scan, to make sure he did not have any blockages in his arteries as he was starting to feel dizzy at random times. He had been to the doctor and his labs were all normal. Well, at that time, I had no idea what to look for, nor did I know any different. His symptoms progressed into abdominal fullness and back pain, but this did not surprise me as he frequently was constipated. The results came back from the scan with some build up in his arteries, but what was more concerning was a spot on his lungs that was seen incidentally. The spot did not shock me as he had smoked for many years. He had quit smoking and had been smoke free at the time of the scan for over four years. It had taken a bout of pancreatitis caused by passing stones from the gallbladder and he was in the hospital for a couple of days, which was unheard of with my very fidgety, busy bodied dad. Corralling him in the hospital was a challenge itself and a whole other story. The following week, he had a scan of his chest completed to further look at the area that was seen in his lungs. The results changed my world forever.

Stage 4 pancreatic cancer that had already spread to his lungs, adrenal glands, liver and prostate. Now, this is a man who felt good overall besides a few episodes of dizziness and abdominal fullness. This man was on the go non-stop. He worked on diesel trucks and was an owner operator of a Semi and delivered flowers. It was his pride and joy. He loved delivering flowers from the greenhouse to the major stores in the area for all of us to shop, buy, plant and enjoy. The reason I tell you all of the background is to help you understand where he was coming from when we saw the oncologist.

With myself being in the medical field and having colleagues to question, I went to several of them asking how this could happen. His labs were wonderful, in fact, the only thing elevated was a prostate screen test, which we were waiting on insurance to get checked out. On his birthday, we sat in the oncologist's office at the cancer institute and she gave him the news. I had already known the news for about a week prior, but knew the news needed to come from the specialist. I had prepared him for bad news, but was fully prepared for him to get a serious slug in the gut when he heard it from a specialist.

It was his 65th birthday when he got the news. I remember watching the color drain from his face. They already had him scheduled for surgical biopsies, chemotherapy and likely radiation as they knew pancreatic cancer was aggressive, and one of the most painful cancers. He was given an estimated 3-6 months to live. He looked at that little gal giving us the news in disbelief and asked her how it was possible that he had all of this and felt good. At first, he was game for everything she was throwing at him for treatment, but when I asked her how much time it would gain him and how he would feel, he quickly changed his mind. Going through the treatment would give him roughly 1-2 more months of life, and he likely would not feel good throughout it. With tears running down his face, he stood up, shook her hand, and said, "I am sorry you have to deliver this kind of news to people. Thank you for your time, we are out of here. I do not want to step foot in a hospital and don't plan to spend any more time here." We were out the door in a flash and in the parking lot when he looked at me and asked me to find another way. He kissed me and said, "I have to go to work," and off he went to haul flowers.

So, I dug into options, did research, and ran across Dr. Kylie Burton's book and quite a few others. At that time, I did not understand what Dr. Kylie was teaching, so her book took a back seat. I treated my father from an all-natural standpoint. We juiced, changed a meat and potatoes man over to all organic everything. Man, that was a challenge, but he had a willpower and spirit that I had never seen. He was eating things he never would have dreamed of and longed for salt and butter and bacon, oh man did he want bacon!

When he started getting weak, I left my job and rode with him in the Semi delivering flowers so I could help load and unload the carts. A loaded cart of flowers is very heavy. I took all of my books, research and literature with me to try to eliminate the nightmare we were given. It was a struggle, you see, being in the truck was his time, his space, pride and joy. As much as he loved me spending time with him, it was hard for him to let me help. During our trips,

I was constantly researching and developing a plan for our next options. He would ask me what I was reading and kept telling me that I needed to continue learning so I could help others. We kept him active and even in the Semi up until 2-3 weeks prior to his passing. While I felt like a failure for not finding him a cure, I was proud that we (my sister, cousin and I) kept him active for so long. He never set foot in the hospital unless he had labs and a repeat scan here or there to see if we were winning or losing. I knew we were losing, but he never lost hope that we were going to beat it. His positivity was endless.

That was my first big jump into supplements and natural health and healing. Mentally, I was struggling and did not know if I could return to work after his passing. I had even considered getting my CDL to drive his Semi and deliver flowers like he did. Then it happened. One morning when I woke up, Dr. Kylie's book was sitting on my chair. I had put it away months before. I asked my husband and my daughters why they had gotten it out and no one fessed up to it. I picked it up, and put it away only to find it back on my chair later that day. So, I re-read it and reached out to her. It just so happened that she had a certification program starting in the next couple of weeks. I choked a little when I invested the money but felt like it was a push from my dad. Within 3 hours of the first class, I had more lightbulbs go off in my head than I had my entire amount of schooling. I knew I was supposed to continue on this path and here I am.

The first moment of victory for me was when I started Dr. Kylie's vitamin D protocol. Within the first ten days, I had more energy, less mood swings and felt better overall. I knew vitamin D was important, but man, did it really make a difference. I now recommend it to everyone, especially those with seasonal depression, anxiety, and fatigue. We live in the northern part of the United States and it now made sense to me that the depletion of vitamin D over the winter months really plays havoc on someone's well-being. Did you know that even people who live in the Caribbean can be deficient in vitamin D? The body needs to be regenerated/rebooted so it can go from unhealthy to healthy and thrive, not just try to survive. The goal for vitamin D is greater than 80. Eighty?! I had never seen it above 34 and had seen it as low as 4! No wonder so many of us feel like garbage. Time to make a change!

Let me provide you with a specialized 90-day program to get your life back so you can join in with your family and friends instead of watching from the sidelines because you don't feel well enough. Maybe that looks like fatigue, depression, anxiety, diarrhea, aches, pains, and on and on, I CAN help you! If you are interested, email me at:

Healthrenovationsllc@gmail.com

Or find me here:

www.tiktok.com/@healthrenovationsllc

https://instagram.com/spohrchantell?igshid=NTc4MTIwNjQ2YQ== https://www.facebook.com/chantell.spohr?mibextid=LQQJ4d

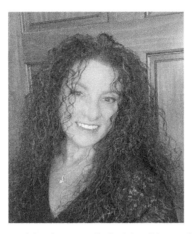

I am a farm/horse girl. I have a little bit of knowledge on a lot of things, so I am a "do it yourself" style person quite frequently. If I don't have my hands in the garden or re-designing a landscape, I am likely into some other project I got myself into. Many times, it starts with a vision that most do not see until it starts coming together. I have a wonderful supportive family and great friends. To say I am blessed, is an understatement.

I never knew what I wanted to do when I grew up, but it all started when I was pregnant with our oldest daughter. I was quite ill and in the emergency room being treated by a wonderful nurse. I wish I knew who she was so I could tell her what she inspired me to do. I signed up for nursing classes that same week. I received my Associates in Nursing as a Registered Nurse in 2007. I started my career in an oncology unit and after a couple of years, transferred to a medical/surgical floor with pediatrics and orthopedics. I stayed there until I had our second daughter. About that time, our oldest was ready to start kindergarten and I found a job closer to home. This job was quite eventful as I was the nurse at the county jail for eight years and man, do I have stories to share with that one. I should write a book. I completed my Bachelors in Nursing and then went on to complete my Masters of Nursing- Family Nurse Practitioner degree in 2017 and have been there since. As a general practitioner, you get a bit of everything and do not specialize in anything, therefore; you don't get the deep depths of any particular area unless you choose to further that knowledge base and education.

I am grateful to have found Dr. Kylie and Mr. Rhees for the knowledge so I can now offer anyone looking for answers, actual answers and solutions! I am still a Family Nurse Practitioner, but stepped into the Health Coach role to help you!

CHAPTER 5:

The Healing Path to Health and Reverse Aging

By: Dr. Kenna S. Ducey-Clark, D.C., P.C.

There is no better time than now.

Everything you have done has led you to where you are at this exact moment. You are reading my words for reasons only you will know. As for me? I'm writing these words because I want to help you. If you happen to be a woman who has been grinding away at life for years, giving, and giving some more, and feeling it in your body, seeing it on your face, experiencing a heaviness in your mind, and your heart is wondering where it's going to muster up the next ounce from; it sounds like now is the time to give a much-needed something back to yourself. If you haven't seen them yet, your body has yellow warning flags flying high with "Help Me" written across them in bright red ink. But guess what? You are reading the right chapter. Or you may be a woman who has experienced that and is presently struggling with some health issues that complicate the needed self-giving, maybe challenges that are so life interfering, you feel lost in chronic illness. In that case, this is the chapter for you too.

This is the chapter for any woman who wants to learn about how providing the body its basic needs well, can lead to positive benefits like helping slow or reverse the aging process and reducing the chances of disease forming. It's also for women who want to learn how to have a better understanding about figuring out what their bodies want and how to attune to its messages sent by signs or signals, what health professionals call "symptoms." This is for any woman who wants to become healthier, or reclaim their health, and it's also for those who feel their health is a lost cause. It is for women who want to learn how to self-advocate for their health and learn what that looks like. Lastly, this chapter is for any woman who is looking for inspiration, maybe some hope, from a true story.

Let me begin with this message that everyone needs to hear sometime in their life. There is no reason why I shouldn't share it with you right now. What your body desires more than anything else is to be *BALANCED*. There, mission accomplished; even if you stop reading right now, you will be walking away with learning something new or being reminded of its importance.

Your body is always working towards being balanced. When your body and all its needed internal systems are operational, being in this state is what scientists call "homeostasis." Your body always wants to do good for you and it's always working to be healthy for you. Try to open your mind to the limitless possibilities of something good happening to your health, despite the things that may or may not have gone wrong. Because even when it is very unwell, it is trying desperately to balance out. It is eagerly waiting for one of those positive possibilities to happen, so it can restore to harmonious homeostasis. This is true even for those whose eyes are reading these words that feel like their body is turning against them. *Trust me; it is not.* It's telling you it's unwell and asking for help. And, for those who are in fabulous health, but are afraid of the day that comes when they aren't, you too need to trust me. Your body is on your side and it needs you to work with it, just like it works with you.

What does this mean and what does this look like? It means that you, like your body, are going to work hard at remaining balanced. If you are on board with working towards balance, welcome to the opportunity to slow or reverse your biological age. This translates into that your biological age is the age of your body and your body's cells. Unlike your chronological age, the number of candles on your birthday cake, aka how many years you have lived, your biological age can REVERSE. YES, a collaborative research study done by Harvard Medical School and Duke Medical School proved that your biological age can be reversed. This study was published in Cell Metabolism May 02, 2023. This is very exciting news! Why? Because this study proves that the damage done to your cells can be repaired. And when those cells are repaired, reversing your biological age is possible. In other words, you can be fifty-five-years-old but have the body of a forty-two-year-old. How? There are many scientists trying to figure that out right now.

The study revealed that SEVERE STRESS increased the acceleration of biological age and disease formation and that biological aging can be reversed, when recovery has occurred. When I read this study, I immediately thought of my happy place, Hawaii. Every time I have visited those islands, it feels and looks like years fall off of my face and inside my body. Within forty-eight hours, the weight of all the unknown stress that I carry, falls aside. You may be wondering what kind of stress this study was talking about. The answer is ALL forms of stress. Physical stress that could be due to an injury, or a needed surgery, exposure to something you are allergic to that's in your living environment, or something that you're allergic to that you eat and put inside your body, toxins, bacteria, fungus, or mold. Stress to your body can be caused by not drinking enough water, not sleeping enough, not eating foods with the proper kind of nutrition, smoking, drinking or eating something in excess, over-exercising, under-exercising, taking the incorrect medications, and the list goes on and on. Stress can also be caused by something that is emotional, like a boss that micromanages, a significant other who is overly critical, money worries, being a caregiver, a traumatic event, parenting, loneliness, low self-esteem, performance pressure, being a people pleaser, being depressed, experiencing long-standing anger, grief, disappointment, etc.

If you are human, you will experience stress in your life. You can't avoid it. But you can be mindful if your stress is severe in nature.

While the research scientists are working on getting hard proof of the specifics of *how* to reverse one's biological age, let's work with what they have already proven and something we understand. Since we now know that severe stress causes biological aging to speed up, what can you do NOW to lessen that impact?

First, commit to solidly giving your body its primary basics NEEDS. What are those?

- Oxygen-breathing
- Sleeping-rest
- Hydration-water
- Nutrition-food
- Exercise-movement

Please, do not skip over this part of my chapter. You'd be surprised how many people are struggling with these basics. Let's begin with your greatest need of all, breathing.

Studies have shown that breath, and how you breathe, can cause premature aging. Literally, being a mouth breather, or someone who breathes shallowly, can negatively impact your immune system, brain, and digestive system. There are many well-known celebrities that have made breathwork a part of their regular daily self-care practice for nervous system calming, anxiety-reducing, energy enhancing, and other positive health benefits: Oprah, Gisele Bundchen, Christy Turlington, and Hailey Bieber.

Who out there is getting a good night of sleep? Sleep can be tricky. In my decades of experience working as a health practitioner, I've crossed paths with thousands of very tired people. I don't know about you, but getting good sleep is extremely impactful to how I will be functioning, or not, the next day. Healthy sleep for women is 7-9 hours a night of uninterrupted, continuous sleep. Healthy sleep increases your mental clarity, helps your mood, regulates your blood sugar, keeps your heart healthy, lowers your stress, and restores your immune system. There really is something to that phrase "getting your beauty sleep." Cellular regeneration in your skin and body occurs when you are sleeping at night. Lots of good and necessary things happen in your body when you are in a deep sleep.

Water, and drinking enough of it, is a challenge for many. There are also volumes of research that link regular hydration with slowing down the aging process and to fending off disease. This comes as no surprise because the average human body is made up of roughly 60% of water.

Proper nutrition- fresh, balanced (lean protein, fresh vegetables and fruits, whole grain, and healthy fats), colorful, nutritious, and non-processed foods, give your body the best chances to reduce accelerated aging.

As for regular exercise, yes, it's been proven in thousands of different ways that it helps humans remain healthy. We are meant to move, not sit.

Evidence shows that all of these basic needs, that we automatically have every day, are proven to prevent accelerated aging and premature disease if done regularly and well. Ask yourself, "Is there something in this group that I can do better with?" If so, I challenge you to grab your smartphone, and in the notes section, type out what you need to improve and how you will do it. Then set a small achievable goal for yourself for the next fourteen days.

The second commitment you need to make is to figure out what your body WANTS. This isn't always easy. It actually can be a little tricky because although one female body is mostly the same as the next, each body has its own unique variances. Figuring out what *your* body wants will take some time and discipline. What the body WANTS can be something to help an already healthy body, or to help a body that is in distress. You'll begin doing this by paying close attention to your body's signals. Track them, use a journal or your notes app. You are looking for a repeating pattern. An example of such is feeling more anxious after a night of six hours of sleep. Or, breaking out with eczema after eating a lot of cheese. You will have to be honest with yourself about what is working for your body and what is not. Maybe eight hours of sleep a night is something your body really wants, not six. Remember, you are aiming to be supportive of all of your body's needs and WANTS, and aiming to eliminate as much stress from its systems as possible. Identifying your body's wants, signals, and patterns is the first step to self-advocating for your health.

Figuring out your body's ideal needs and wants will require attention and action. It will lead you down the path that will come to a crossroads. This is where you'll choose to change or stay the same.

Did I just lose you right there, when I mentioned the word C-H-A-N-G-E? When something isn't working or you want to make something better than it already is, you will need to change something. Change and changes can lead you to some really good things. I know this because I've been helping people make good changes that positively impact their level of health for decades and

I, too, have had to make changes myself. When changing feels challenging below are two things, I remind people of to help them stay motivated:

- *What you put into your body is most likely what you are going to get out of it.*
- *Your body, that beautiful vessel that is your forever home, wants to make you happy, wants you to feel healthy, and wants you to thrive in your life. What are you willing to do to help it?*

Your body is your one and only home for your entire lifetime. Don't be afraid of it! You are capable of learning its quirks and what works for it and what doesn't, without being a health professional. You don't need to have a Ph.D. in Biochemistry, be an expert in anatomy, or understand the intimidating medical language health professionals speak to know your body. You are the sole owner of that vessel. It is 100% yours. Treat it like its value—a multi-million-dollar property. Care for it, nourish it, and love it. If it has issues that lead to seeking professional health advice or care, DO NOT relinquish ownership. Self-advocate for your health. Your healthcare professional is in the business to care for your health. Try not to make assumptions that the information you have about your body will not be valid because you are speaking to a specialist. Share what you know about your body's truth. Ask questions, take notes, and if things don't add up for you then get a second opinion, and maybe even a third. Listen to your gut. That first instinct you have tells you a lot. I remember what my gut said when I first met the surgeon that I shouldn't have chosen. I also remember what my gut said when my case was reviewed by another surgeon after a past surgery outcome was not optimal. He looked me dead straight in the eyes and said, "Do not go back to this surgeon." I didn't. Try not to override your gut instinct. Listen to your inner voice. It is wise.

In the not-so-far past, I remember the exact moment I felt myself walking away from "the old me." That's what I refer to myself when talking about the time in my life when I, the picture of health and an expert in the health field, nonetheless became very ill. My health forecast back then, what we doctors call a "prognosis," looked like the Titanic heading straight toward the iceberg. Like the Titanic at the beginning of its voyage, I looked and felt unsinkable before I got sick. I was in the prime of my life, fit, full of energy, looking and feeling years younger than my actual age. I was many things. A wife, mother, doctor, and friend, who was living a beautiful life. Back then I happily ran my successful integrative clinic, which had been operating for close to two decades. I worked in the field of professional sports my entire career. So, part of my daily routine was to care for a champion or two and often a champion's family member. At that time, my job was "championing for champions." Doing this well required not only my expertise and decades of training but also dedication to delivering a level of health care that exceeded expectations to my patients AND to myself. I ate a clean diet, was in the Pure Barre studio five days a week, rode the Peloton, and regularly walked if I wasn't jogging. My healthy lifestyle delivered results.

I'm a goal-oriented person by nature. Just like I did for my patients, I created a manageable plan for myself that was sustainable and easy to follow. This was highly motivating. I set small achievable goals and by following those consistently, I was golden. Much like the Titanic before it left port, I had my health and health routine polished up so well it shined. I suspected the same way that ship did as it moved through the icy waters of the Atlantic. So, I thought.

With each step, I felt my heart rate hold steady. I heard my running shoes rhythmically hitting the payment with an even beat. It felt so good to move my body once again, pain-free. At that moment, I felt pure exhilaration. Joyful tears streamed down my cheeks as I realized I was going to be OK. Then it hit me; I was going to be much better than OK; I was going to be the healthy version of myself that, at times, I thought was lost forever. I was back, and "the old me" was gone.

As I began breathing more heavily, and my speed increased, I began thinking about how the past few years felt like a bad dream, a nightmare. That's when the chronic illness began knocking at my door due to a necessary surgery that didn't go as planned. The risks that came with the surgery, far outweighed the risks of not getting it. But I didn't think I'd be one of the unlucky few to fall in the percentile of the unfortunate. When the surgery reconstruction began to fail inside, my body literally began to fall apart, my immune system's reaction went into high kill alert. The white blood cells that make up my body's internal defense army started attacking everything, destroying whatever was in its path, thousands upon thousands of my healthy cells. This is what happens when you experience autoimmune disease. Self attacks self. This means your immune cells that are meant to fend off things in your body like viruses or bacteria, instead attack your healthy cells. That's when I, who had always been the doctor, became the official patient.

Prior to that surgery, my body gave me plenty of warning signals that let me know it was struggling to stay in a balanced state. The first sign I noticed was my energy was slightly lower. I wasn't as peppy as my usual self. It was so subtle I didn't notice it when it was happening at the time. But as I began retracing my health decline, I remembered feeling a little more labored in my Pure Barre classes that I normally buzzed through that September. I knew it was normal for my body to have energy and endurance cycles and shifts, so I shook it off. The next signal was a change in my skin. It lost its normal luster. I have skin that naturally glows and that October it became very flat. I invested in facial serums that helped a little, but the results were temporary. I focused more on the products than on why my skin was acting up. This was a big miss on my part.

As a practitioner, I always paid close attention to skin health. I'd often explained to my patients, "your skin is the largest organ your body has. When there is an underlying problem within the body, the first noticeable traces of an issue will often show up in the skin. Eczema, acne of all kinds, and psoriasis are indicators that something isn't right in the body, not just with the skin but somewhere else." Sometimes you really can't see the forest from the trees. Remember, I was doing everything that you should do to remain healthy and I was the picture of health. I wrote off the lack of luster because of the change of seasons. That early December I awoke one morning feeling like all my energy had been sucked out of me. I knew my clinic schedule was booked solid that day and I needed to get going. I sat up on the side of my bed with difficulty. I felt random pain all over my body, I braced my thighs with my hands trying to push myself up to a vertical position. I wasn't going anywhere, at least for a few minutes. As I sat slumped on the side of the bed, I did a self-evaluation. "What are you feeling, Dr. Ducey-Clark?" I whispered to myself. I felt like there were a million shards of glass floating in my body, and the energy I went to bed with the night before, was secretly sucked out of me by a Hoover vacuum. I was so tired. All I wanted to do was lay back down in bed. But that wasn't an option, so I thought. "I've got to go to work," I said to myself, taking in a big inhale. With the exhale, I stood up, pushing through the discomfort, and dug deep into my body's reserves. There was work to be done. This was the day that I began paying attention to my symptoms. Those subtle signals had turned into full-blown symptoms.

Seeing patterns in the health of my patients was as easy as breathing to me. I'd connect dots of their body's subtle signs, look at the symptoms, history and labs, and they'd always lead me to reasons, and causes of why they were experiencing issues in their health. I knew pain was not the first signal the body would give out, unless there was a blunt-force injury, like a stubbed toe. The kind of pain I was experiencing came far after many non-painful signals were sent out. This was the day that I learned I was human just like the rest of the world. "I am not a superhero. Do not panic," I wrote in my first journal that I began tracking the signs and symptoms. I kept food journals, mood journals, and journals of all kinds, keeping a close eye on the daily patterns of my health and lifestyle. I knew my health history, as well as my family's, and I was looking for something to help me better understand why my body was sending distress signals. I began doing something for myself that I had done thousands of times for others - single out a problem-causing pattern.

There are many studies that support the theory that humans are creatures of habit all the way to the cellular level. What does this mean? You have repeating patterns that you do over and over again all the way down to your single cellular level. Do you know how many cells make up your body? 37.2 trillion cells! It's crazy, but it is true. We are a bit of a broken record, all 37.2 trillion cells that is.

Are all of these cells doing the same thing? No, but there's a lot of repetitive behaviors happening that's for sure. Sometimes the broken record, aka patterns, become unhealthy because they need to change. At other times, patterns get disrupted because of unhealthy influences. This may be one of the reasons why change is so hard for us. A funny thing about change is it is one of the few guarantees that comes with living a human life. You unknowingly have changes occurring in your body every second. Each day that passes is filled with changes, and the day that comes after today, tomorrow, will bring with it a guaranteed change. You will be one day older. Changes are happening so often that we don't even notice them. And still, we resist change.

I was born with the unique ability to identify patterns that are often overlooked or unseen by others. I have been this way as far back as I can remember. I can detect subtleties in the tone of voice, see a slight change in someone's complexion, easily identify the variance in the way someone walks, notice the shift in eating patterns, sleeping patterns, speaking patterns, emotional patterns, and the list goes on and on. As I began maturing in life, so did my curiosity to understand why the patterns were occurring. It was much like connecting the dots. I would see a cause or multiple causes, that would lead to a result. For example, decades ago I noticed that one of my high school friends always got a terrible stomach ache, which was followed by a full day of horrible anxiety the day after she ate a jelly donut. I noticed weird things that people didn't see with ease. As I aged, I wanted to understand why things like this were happening and how to help them from not happening again. What I wanted was to be a doctor.

My desire to serve others, combined with this innate ability, were core reasons why I pursued a career in health. First, I wanted to go to medical school. I wanted to work in the field of pediatrics and considered being a surgeon. But then I recognized my passion was finding a way to incorporate alternative health approaches with traditional care. I desired to learn about practices that focused on the health of not only the physical body, but also those that took into account the emotional and spiritual influences on health too. I wanted to learn about holistic health care. So, I decided that chiropractic school would be a better fit for me than medical school. Shortly after I began studying to be a doctor of chiropractic, I learned that like the medical doctors, they didn't follow a holistic approach either. I remained in chiropractic school, although I strongly considered changing my course and heading back to medical school. I found my way and have no regrets about my path. Through years of training, I met professors, researchers, and other doctors that provided additional educational sources to help me fine-tune my understanding of holistic health. While in chiropractic school I fell in love with nutrition, learned my brain understood biomechanics and found my place in the field of sports medicine, and discovered a new health approach called Functional Medicine. Function Medicine was a concept that I could get behind. Those doctors who believed in the philosophy of functional medicine looked for the cause of the health problems while addressing the symptoms. This is unlike traditional medicine which is all about treating symptoms alone. So, over twenty-five years ago I aligned with the functional medicine approach, followed a holistic health philosophy, and began incorporating that with my chiropractic training. Not many were doing this, and a day in my clinic often looked like this.

One day I walked into one of my treatment rooms to find an enormous man draped over the treatment table. To protect his identity, I've changed some of the specifics of this story, and will refer to him as "Bear." Bear looked like a giant rhinoceros laying on a picnic table bench. His size and presence dwarfed the room. The still body of this pro athlete became instantly alive when I heard a deep raspy voice say, "Doc is that you? Don't mind me. I'm taking a nap and a break from this pain. I'm dying here. It feels like I have a knife in my side. No one helps this except you. Do your magic." Even though he's talking face down into a treatment table his voice resonates through the room like he's on a megaphone. This man has a commanding presence, on and off the field. I'll admit he is intimidating. But I quickly learned early on working with him, that underneath his façade of being a human steamroller, feared by many, he was a gentle giant. I responded to Bear in a sing-song way, "yes sir, it is I. Nap time is over. Will you please sit up so we can talk about what's going on?" What was going on was the million-dollar question.

Bear had fractured a rib in the previous season which had fully healed, without any complications. And yet, he kept experiencing recurrent painful "flare ups" that were interfering with the quality of his life and his livelihood, aka how he played in his games. It was off-season and his body was in rest mode. The usual daily trauma that it had become accustomed to wasn't occurring. He was following my orders, giving himself some much-needed rest. Yet still, there he was laying down in my clinic, feeling exhausted by his pain. I pulled up recent X-Rays, and looked at his MRI. They were both normal. I moved to his blood panel reports, all were normal, actually extremely healthy, with one exception, his C-Reactive Protein (CRP). "Ah-hah," I whispered to myself. CRP is a protein that is made by the liver. When it increases, it is a marker that indicates there is inflammation in your body. Testing for CRP is most commonly used by heart doctors, cardiologists, looking for heart disease. I use this test panel often to flag if there is a presence of inflammation caused by infection, a chronic inflammatory disease, or an autoimmune disease. I then said, "I understand that you are hurting. Is there anything else that's been happening with your body that seems unusual? Have you made any changes to your diet? Or have you added anything new to your supplement routine?" He paused for a moment and then answered while questioning his memory, "You know something hasn't been right with my BM's. I didn't bring it up because I didn't think you'd want to hear about it." I shook my head and said, "Anything that is related to your health I want to hear about. What's going on with your BM's? How long has this been happening and have you changed anything in your diet?"

Long story short, this man met the love of his life ten months earlier and she was an excellent cook. She began making him homemade pasta to help his carb load. He loved it so much; he ate her pasta sometimes up to five days a week. This is when his issues with stomach cramping began, his bowel movements became increasingly runny, diarrhea, and more frequent. At the same time, his old rib fracture spot began hurting him like it was newly injured. "You know doc, I used to eat rice before I met her. I only like pasta that is super fresh, like it tastes in Italy. Now she makes it for me all the time." I ordered more tests and one came back positive. He had Celiac disease.

Celiac is an autoimmune disease that primarily affects the gut, often the small intestine. People with Celiac disease develop an intolerance to foods containing gluten. Gluten is a sticky protein found in foods like wheat, rye, and barley. Wheat flour was the main ingredient of his homemade pasta. He had been consuming foods with gluten in it his entire life. But admittedly, shared that before the homemade pasta, he was avoiding many foods that had a high gluten content in them. He told me that he hated beer and stopped drinking it because it made him bloated. "I've been fine my entire life. Why is this Celiac happening now?" he asked. "Bear, from the sounds of it, Celiac has been happening to you most of your life. You've shared you've had issues with stomach bloating since you were in high school and have been avoiding foods that made you feel unwell. Your body was sending out signals for years that you didn't register as true symptoms of an underlying issue. You were pretty stressed out by the rib fracture, and had a very challenging season before you began to eat all that homemade pasta. At that time your body was experiencing both physical stress from the injury and emotional stress from that crazy season. STRESS tipped your immune system to move in the wrong direction and your immune system got very confused. It's all connected, your physical health, your emotions, and also how you feel spiritually. Your body is a little out of balance. Don't worry, there are ways to calm everything down, help reduce your pain, and get your gut healthier."

I understood Celiac and sensitivities to gluten very well and assured him that I would guide him back to feeling 110% once again. The first step was eliminating the main culprit to his problem, all gluten-containing foods. Now there are strong opinions about gluten and eliminating foods completely from the diet. With Celiac Disease, the way to calm the autoimmune response is to remove gluten. There's no way around it. I know many people that have Celiac that still eat foods with gluten. But I do not encourage it. If gluten is a trigger to cause an autoimmune reaction, then I say don't eat it. This champion agreed with my guidance and without hesitation removed gluten from his diet that day! After one week, he lost seven pounds and his pain was beginning to go away. I knew he needed some extra support so I gave him a pharmaceutical-grade nutritional supplementation plan to follow. This three-month plan was designed to help calm, replenish, and restore. He resumed beginning his day with a fifteen-minute daily meditation to help clear his mind and manage his stress, and added in flow yoga two times a week to his strict training program. In a matter of weeks, his stomach stopped hurting, his pain went away, his bowel movements became normal, he lost fifteen pounds without trying and his energy returned. He was vertical once again.

Fast forward years later, I found myself in my own spiraling health situation. After my third surgery with non-optimal results, my body was sending out many warning signals. This is when the surgical reconstruction began to fail inside of me. I recall looking at my reflection in the bathroom mirror and seeing a mere shadow of myself staring back. "What is happening to you?" I asked. Do you know what it feels when your body is acting in a way that you don't understand? What a silly question. Of course, you do. That's why you are reading this. When this was occurring, it was in the early months of the COVID pandemic. It was pure chaos in the world and especially in the world of healthcare. I, an experienced doctor, who understood the body's inner workings, found myself overtaken by the COVID tsunami that swept over many who needed healthcare that wasn't related to that virus. Because of the restriction imposed to slow COVID, I wasn't able to access the care I needed. I determined it was safer for me to stay home than to be hospitalized. Confident and determined that I would heal myself from my bed with my laptop, I dug into boatloads of research. My love for data fueled my desire to collect as much information as I could. I strongly believe that information often leads to empowerment. I teach this to my patients regularly. "You are scared of the unknown," I compassionately told a frightened patient. "Let's fill that unknown space with knowledge. Knowledge is empowerment." When I felt my fear creep in, I dove into books, combed through decades of research, reached out to colleagues and their colleagues; I called researchers, and then when able, knocked on doors, and waited in waiting rooms all day to take the place of someone who decided not to show up for their appointment. I did everything I could to figure out what was happening to my body. This is what self-advocacy looked like for me. I wasn't going to go down without a fight.

I continued on my steady run and my memories flooded my mind. I often questioned how people without the training I had, or education, survive what I just survived? What I went through was unthinkable. Never in my wildest dreams did I imagine this experience would be a part of my life story. But it was. It was a chapter in my life story. I'm only giving it a chapter because I won't allow it any more space. I'm hopeful that the space that it does fill, helps someone else in a difficult chapter in their life. I continued to move down the road as my least favorite chapter began unfolding inside my head.

When I was a small child, I experienced a traumatic event. It was super scary for my little self and despite my courage and ability to recover, I'm fairly certain that was the first time my immune system was shocked. Severe stress of any form, physical, emotional, and even spiritual can open the floodgates within the body and cause an inflammatory storm. An inflammatory storm is when the immune system, specifically the white blood cells that create an internal cellular army meant to fend off invaders, such as unwanted viruses, bacteria, parasites, fungus, and anything else that shouldn't be there, go a little crazy. This kind of severe stress can activate something within the cellular matrix, and at times, may cause the cellular army to get confused and start attacking its own healthy cells. After my early childhood trauma, whenever I got stressed, my little body responded with stomach aches that were so bad I would fall to the ground in pain. I don't know when the swelling began, swelling of my entire body that is. To this day, swelling is one of the first warning signs my body gives when I am having a reaction to anything unfavorable. I clearly remember sitting in my kindergarten class and feeling the seams of my dress cut into my armpit when my body began blowing up like a balloon. My mother would take me to doctors and they'd either say it was a virus or that I was "sensitive." And sometimes they'd say they couldn't find evidence of anything being wrong.

 When I was a kid, stomachaches were normal. And issues with health in little ones were uncommon. I knew kids that were allergic to bees, a few that had an allergy to milk and "grew out of it", and a couple of unlucky kids that were deathly allergic to peanuts. There were no fat-free, gluten-free, lactose-free products anywhere. Everyone ate what was available, including me. My parents were health-conscious and fed us a well-balanced diet full of fresh, whole, non-processed foods, loaded with lean meats, healthy fats, fruits, and vegetables. There were no Pop Tarts, Wonder Bread, or Fruit Loops in our pantry ever. Despite the healthy food, I was still sick often. In hindsight, I was sick when I felt stressed. And, the symptoms I experienced were continually written off by doctors as a stomach virus, food poisoning, or because I was deemed "sensitive." If I had counted, I bet I experienced "food poisoning" thousands of times in my childhood. What would my "food poisoning" look like? It always included terrible painful bloating, irregular bowel movements, horrible diarrhea, and vomiting. I know, TMI. Trust me it wasn't pretty. The worst part for me, besides the pain in my gut, was the bloating and swelling. Now, I'm not a petite human. I stand 5' 10" tall and was always one of the tallest, if not the tallest, girls in my class growing up. So even when I'm very healthy, I am not small. But the bloating and swelling at any given time easily added a good 15 pounds of inflammation to my body. I hated this! The discomfort that resulted from carrying the extra weight was awful. But the accusations by others that I over-ate and under-exercised were torturous. I did neither. As a result, I under-ate and over-exercised. Which as a result caused stress, the worst thing for my immune system.

Well before I knew I wanted to be a doctor of any kind, I began tracking my signs and symptoms. Slowly but surely, I figured out what made me sick and what made me feel well. Common foods I'd ingest like white flour products, bread, baked goods, and pasta and things in my physical environment such as strong chemical agents, paint thinner, ant spray and cleaning agents, aggravated my body, causing exaggerated painful symptoms. I began removing everything that I reacted to out of my diet and from my home, and my symptoms became less and less. Much to my amazement, the weight began falling off without an effort. My pain started to lessen, my bowel movements began to become more regular, my skin cleared, and my energy increased. I believe my own highly sensitive immune system helped seed my compassion for others who were suffering, and eventually led to a passion for clinical nutrition, my alignment with the holistic health philosophy, and fueled my quest to find an alternate health approach to care, in lieu of traditional medicine health practices.

My feet kept moving and I was much farther from home than I planned. I was working out the hard life chapter once and for all. I recalled thinking about Bear often when I was on my own health journey. He had done everything right when it came to his health for most of his life. His health resources were top-notch, and his body was everything that a champion's should be. His body worked masterfully and could do things others could not. And, then he met the love of his life and she made some wicked homemade pasta. Because she loved him so very much, she made him a lot of that pasta and then things went sideways for Bear. Who would have ever thought that pasta made because of love, would lead to Bear's mini-health crisis? I had a lot in common with this champion. No, I wasn't a professional athlete, but I had a similar lifestyle, a woman's midlife version, and had the best health resources. I thought of Bear's story because I was looking for my body's equivalent to Bear's pasta.

Autoimmune disease can be cruel and very painful, especially when untreated. The physical and emotional stress of five surgeries sent my immune system into overdrive. After the final surgery was a great success, I waited for my body to bounce back. I was ready to return back to my life, but it didn't bounce back. The fatigue continued, as did the brain fog and pain in my gut. I was past the normal recovery time and knew something was very wrong. I went back to more doctors, who didn't have any answers to why I was still struggling. One asked me if I was depressed. My jaw almost dropped to the floor when I heard that question. "Do you know who I am and what my training is? No, I am not depressed. I am sick and want your advice on the next steps to take so I can get better." I answered with restraint and calm, despite my disbelief I was asked this question. Another inferred that I wasn't feeling what

I was feeling. Doctors are humans, and sometimes they have human moments. Almost all of my doctors and caregivers were amazing. I wouldn't be here writing this if it hadn't been for them. Yet still, I had to self-advocate for myself the entire time. When it was inferred my symptoms weren't real, I feared I'd get trapped in a loophole of inadequacy and never fully recover. I took matters into my own hands and ordered some blood panels for myself. I told my husband, "I know there is something wrong with my body. I ordered labs because I need answers. We're paying for these tests out of pocket." My husband was my rock and agreed emphatically with my decision.

He was taking a nap on a Friday afternoon when the blood panels came in. I opened the labs like it was Christmas morning, hoping to see something that would help me help myself. The markers indicated infection, severe adrenal fatigue, and an immune system that was on fire with an autoimmune disease. I waited in a chair in front of our bed for one hour until his eyes opened up. As soon as they did I calmly said, "I know what is wrong with me. I know how to fix this and I know what to do." I was so excited, I explained to him the significance of the blood panels, the markers that I flagged, and what I was going to do to help myself. In that moment my fear of being forever sick was replaced with absolute relief. I was a specialist who understood how to calm an immune system that was on fire. Yes, my body experienced a lot of traumas while it went through all of those surgeries, and now it was having an autoimmune reaction fallout. It was impacting multiple systems in my body. I looked at my lab results with hearts in my eyes. Remember, I replace fear with information. I took that information and ran with it.

As I turned back towards home, I felt the adrenaline kick in, my body loosen, and came to the clear realization that my crazy experience had begun with stress. Stress was my equivalent to

Bear's pasta. And like for Bear, I created a similar plan for myself to help my body restore, replenish, rebalance, and heal. I used nutritional supplementation, diet, and lifestyle modifications to help my body have an epic comeback. My recovery did not happen overnight, or even in a few months - it took a full year. But with each day, I made improvements and was better than I was the day before. With the recovery, I began to reverse aging. I kid you not. As my body regulated and began functioning optimally, my energy and focus returned, my pain lessened, the lines on my face started disappearing, and the glow in my skin was revived. As the severe stress lessened in my life, my cells began to recover and regenerate. Just like the study the Harvard and Duke Medical Schools proved. It was cellular perfection!

When my body gave the first warning signs before it needed any kind of surgery, the signs I shrugged off as nothing, I was doing a lot of things right to keep myself healthy, but I was also doing something wrong. This is where the honesty of my own self-reflection comes in. Yes, at that time I was the picture of health. Yes, my healthstyle and lifestyle were pretty darn good. But I overlooked one very important fact, and that was I was burning my proverbial candle from the top, bottom, and center. I was being everything for everyone. Women do this to themselves. I was over-exerting, and pushing myself beyond my physical limitations until my immune system tipped. Then I pushed some more and my body broke. Why? Because severe stress has always been my Achilles heel since I was a small child.

I believe everything happens for a reason. Even hard lessons like my off-roading health crisis experience. Wow, was that a painful journey, but an incredibly valuable one too. What I learned was I needed to practice what I preached. I thought I was. Balance is key. Balance needs to be healthy even when you are following healthy practices. I was reminded that health is not always linear, nor is it as black and white as most think. It is layered in shades of gray, and comes with chances of twists and turns even the most prepared and experienced may not anticipate. Going through these experiences brought to my attention that women's health didn't become a primary interest for medical and health care agencies until the 1990's. That wasn't very long ago ladies. We've been riding in the back seat for centuries when it comes to health care. I admit, I felt this during my journey. Because of this I learned how to use my voice differently, to self-advocate like my life depended on it, because it did. I also learned how to ask for help, to say "no", and to lean into my family and inner circle, just like they had my entire life. Yes, there were many reasons why this happened to me. I feel the most important reason of all, was the experience gave me a clearer understanding of how to better help women.

When I made it home, I stood in front of my house mindfully slowing my heart rate and catching my breath. Gosh, it felt great to be in a healthy body once again. This is when the idea of HEALTHSTYLE by Dr. Kenna, LLC first came to my mind. "How can I help and motivate women to have a better understanding and relationship with their health?" I asked myself. In the next phase of my career, I wanted to use my knowledge, expertise, and experience to be channeled in a way that would have a positive IMPACT on women collectively. Everything in my life had changed, and in that process, I changed too. My days of being a traditional clinician had come to an end. I wanted to reach more people, and I wanted to work with women specifically. Over the decades of working in health care, I observed that women's relationship with their health was often abstract. I thought about the world and those who've become female role models and wondered where the healthy female role models are. Oprah was the only thought leader that came to mind that talked about her health. Women do it all these days, partner, parent, work, birth babies, raise kids, care for aging parents, organize, clean, cook, make, provide, innovate, generate and so much more. How to do this was never discussed in health education. Yes, we've seen female leaders, celebrities, and supermodels appear perfect, effortlessly having it all together. Perfect doesn't exist in our human experience. What was really happening behind the façade of perfection?

Health isn't only about the physical, but also the emotional health, and the health of our heart's true wants, desires, and will, our soul. It is all connected. I remember patients coming into my clinic every year at the same time (holiday season), with the same physical pain, and with the same emotional strain occurring. Our whole health, the full package, dramatically influences our aging process and ability to prevent disease. Were the health and beauty industries letting women know about this, I questioned? Introducing a new health concept for women to engage with their health that invoked motivation, self-care, and inspiration, in positive evolving ways, was my future. I was tired of being in the backseat when it came to my health, I knew other women felt the same. Nor did I appreciate that as women age it was unfavorable when for men it's quite the opposite. This is when I pivoted into the world of Health and Wellness coaching. Using scientific research, my functional medicine approach combined with a holistic health philosophy, I began creating plans to help women optimize their health and aging process, slow or reverse their biological age, and style their health. Helping women formulate their own unique Healthstyle identity, successfully aided them to engage and relate with their health in an entirely new way. I've watched women blossom into the best version of themselves by nurturing their health and choosing their ideal Healthstyle.

I have created a free downloadable mini-course that is available to you to learn how to identify your unique Healthstyle. It also provides helpful steps and tips on how you can begin editing your health today that will lead to impactful results. If you are interested in taking advantage of this, please head to my website www.HEALTHSTYLEBYDRKENNA.com to sign up for the mini-course. I also work with a select few one-on-one clients and offer a limited number of complimentary fifteen-minute consultations for those who are ready to make some serious Healthstyle changes that will be offered on my website also.

If you've made it this far into my chapter, I hope you believe that I can see you. How you are feeling, and how you engage with your health really matters to me. I understand what it is like to be many things, a woman who is healthy, unhealthy, getting healthier, and becoming healthy once again. Let me finish the same way I began and remind you that the thing your body wants more than anything else is to be balanced and healthy for you. What you put into your body is what you'll get out of it. The quality of your body's basic needs is impactful, as is understanding its wants. There are limitless possibilities for you and your health, no matter what. Investing energy and effort into your Healthstyle pays off. I hope my chapter has helped you and instilled the belief that anything is possible…ANYTHING.

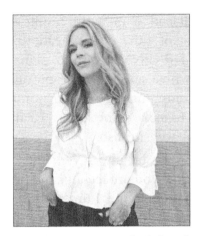

For decades, **Dr. Kenna S. Ducey-Clark** has helped thousands reconnect with and heal themselves, enabling them to go from a surviving state to a thriving state of wellness. An expert in holistic health, trained Doctor of Chiropractic, Functional Medicine practitioner, Health and Wellness Coach, and published author, her career began in sports medicine, utilizing a mechanical application. Recognizing the impact of physiological, mental, and spiritual aspects with performance recovery, her care approach uniquely evolved, integrating holistic, traditional health, and alternative health practices. Her passion for women's health has become the forefront of her life's work and she works with women from around the world. She happily resides in Denver, CO with her husband, daughter, and faithful rescue dog.

CHAPTER 6:

It's Not Your Thyroid

By: Dr. Mark R. Shane, D.C.

"**I**'m tired. All the time."

Beth, a thirty-six-year-old mother of three told me it was hard to remember the last time she felt well. "Maybe in my mid-twenties," she said, but since the birth of her first, her energy started to decline. Not that she hadn't been looking for answers. She went to her doctor who told her everything looked good on her labs and to try and get more rest. She went online and read blogs about constant fatigue and tried changing her diet, exercise, and adding meditation and yoga. Her medicine cabinet was filled with bottles of supplements that had helped others. Her doctor told her that since her mother and older sister had thyroid issues, she would likely need to be on medication at some point. "It's in your family history," she was told, and you can't change that.

At a checkup a few years ago, her doctor said that he had found her problem. She had high TSH. Her thyroid gland was not producing enough hormone so she needed to take a replacement hormone to supplement what her own thyroid couldn't produce. Finally! She had an answer. It was a relief to know she wasn't going to have to live this way for the rest of her life. She immediately filled the prescription and started taking her medication.

Three months later on her check-up visit, her doctor proudly announced that her TSH was now normal. "Then why don't I feel any better? Why is my skin still dry and my constipation has not improved. My hair is still falling out and it takes me forever to get to sleep at night." "Let's adjust the dosing of your medication and give it some more time," said her doctor.

Six months later she returned to her doctor. Her labs were perfect. The medication was working. "Hang in there and you should be feeling better soon."

As she sat in my office, she explained that she barely managed to get through her work day as an administrative assistant. When she got home, it was all she could do to get dinner on the table. Weekends were all about getting rested up enough to face Monday morning again. There was nothing left over for all the fun things she used to enjoy. She reluctantly admitted that she must be suffering from depression because her doctor had given her a mood elevating drug on her last visit.

"You are not alone in this," I explained. I had heard her story hundreds of times. Years of not feeling well but labs were "normal". At least from a standard medical perspective.

What vs. Why?

The What: fatigue, hair loss, low libido, constipation, dry skin, brittle nails, weight gain/weight loss resistance, cold hands and feet, depression, brain fog, joint and muscle aches, irregular periods...and more.

The Why?: The standard medical answer is that the thyroid isn't producing enough hormone. When that happens, the pituitary gland (a small master gland in the brain) increases the level of TSH, thyroid stimulating hormone. But the thyroid can't answer the call so the thyroid keeps asking the pituitary to make more hormone but driving up TSH levels, while T3, the active form of thyroid hormone, stays low. No problem. The doctor prescribes a synthetic thyroid hormone, usually Synthroid or levothyroxine. Now the pituitary sees there is enough thyroid hormone so TSH lowers and the blood work now looks normal.

Sometimes this works great in terms of relieving symptoms. At least for a while and rarely long term. So, if hormone replacement isn't the answer, what do you do?

That is what Beth asked me during our consultation. Why is my energy still in the tank along with all these other symptoms yet my doctor says my labs are normal? If frustration were money, all my thyroid patients would be rich.

It's Not Your Thyroid

What Beth didn't know is that for the great majority of hypothyroid sufferers, the problem is not the thyroid and that taking the hormone replacement drugs has zero chance of fixing the problem! Around ninety percent of hypothyroid is really an autoimmune condition called Hashimoto's Thyroiditis. This is why standard medical care never gets to a solution.

Autoimmunity means your immune system, designed to attack and kill invading microbes, is attacking your tissues instead. In the case of Hashimoto's, your immune system is hard at work trying to kill your thyroid! Sooner or later, the immune system's attack will win and your thyroid will be so damaged it must be removed. Some of you may already be there. Your thyroid was removed and you must take hormone replacement for the rest of your life.

This does not mean however that you are ok and that there is nothing more to do. Autoimmunity is a mechanism. We give autoimmune diseases names based on the tissue under attack. Hashimoto's if it's thyroid. Rheumatoid arthritis if it's the joints in your hands. Multiple sclerosis if it's your nervous system. The list goes on to include celiac, type 1 diabetes, psoriasis, scleroderma,

Guillain-Barre, Grave's disease. There are more than 100 in all. There is no rule that says your autoimmune condition can only attack one tissue. Just because your thyroid is gone doesn't mean you are well.

Autoimmunity is a mechanism with dozens of manifestations. Think of it like this. Baskin-Robbins is an ice cream store and it has thirty-one flavors.

The test for Hashimoto's is an expanded thyroid blood panel that includes the thyroid antibodies TPO and TGA, not just the pituitary hormone TSH that is the only thyroid marker typically looked at. Usually, thyroid antibodies are not tested unless you are sent to a rheumatologist, a doctor specializing in autoimmune diseases. Once this test comes back positive, you finally have your medical diagnosis.

When I explained this to Beth she said, "oh, I forgot to tell you. I have been to the specialist and she checked my thyroid antibodies. I have Hashimoto's. I didn't think to mention it because the doctor said there was no treatment for autoimmune thyroid disease beyond what I was already doing by taking the hormone replacement drugs." I believe this is likely why most doctors don't test for the antibodies. It wouldn't make a difference in treatment so why bother. Besides, who wants to sit in front of a patient and explain you have a disease that they have no treatment for.

So, if Hashimoto's autoimmune thyroid disease is the WHAT, let's ask WHY.

There are about a dozen common drivers of the autoimmune mechanism:
- General infections (mold, parasites, Lyme, virus, bacteria)
- Leaky gut/Microbiome dysbiosis
- Heavy metals (mercury, lead, aluminum, etc.)
- Toxic chemicals (pesticides, herbicides, preservatives,

flame retardants; 80,000+)
- Nutritional deficiencies
- Diet (pro-inflammatory diet/Standard American Diet [SAD])
- Vitamin D deficiency
- Genetics (MTHFR gene for example)
- Gluten intolerance
- Food sensitivities
- Insulin surges
- Hormone imbalance/estrogen surges/perimenopause/menopause
- GI infections
- Iodine (excess)

Almost everything on this list causes inflammation.

The next WHY question to be answered is about inflammation. We have known for many years that inflammation drives all chronic degenerative disease from arthritis to Alzheimer's and everything in between, including hypothyroid. Great, we have our answer now, right? Not quite.

The fact that inflammation leads to degenerative disease is not news. We have known this for decades. Several years back, a national magazine cover proclaimed this fact and contained a long article making the scientific case for how inflammation causes so many problems. Near the end of the article was a section on what to do about it. You are going to like this…the article concludes that since inflammation is the culprit, science needs to develop more and better anti-inflammatory drugs. Are you kidding me?! How about you and I ask one more WHY question.

What is driving inflammation? And, what is going on to hinder the body's ability to handle inflammation? Now we are getting somewhere!

The basic blood work you already have is loaded with these answers. You just have to know how to read it. For example, if your CBC (complete blood count) shows your neutrophils (a type of white blood cell) are over 60%, you have a low grade bacterial and/or fungal infection. If another white blood cell type, your lymphocytes, are above 30%, you have a viral infection. There are more blood markers to look at but you get the point. If you have an infection, you automatically have inflammation and inflammation is damaging your thyroid. Go take a look at your most recent labs. In fact, go look at as many past labs as you can find. You may be surprised at how long you have been fighting this hidden enemy that you didn't even know existed.

How many doses of Levothyroxine does it take to handle a hidden infection in your body? Wrong question, right? No wonder your TSH reads normal yet you still feel like crap. This is just one example of what your blood work can tell us about the root of your condition.

Finding answers to the WHY is the hard part. The easy part is something built into each one of us. That is the ability to heal. This is a free gift baked into our DNA.

Our bodies were designed by God to be self-healing. Period.

So, if this is true, why are you still sick? Another good question. Let me explain with an analogy.

True or false question: on its own, water flows downhill? True. Now, one day I go out and build a dam. I stopped the water from flowing. Second question. Choose A or B. I go out and remove the dam. Do I (A) need to coax, encourage, invite or direct the water to start flowing again or (B) get the heck out of the way?! Exactly. It's B. It just flows by itself because of the natural law of gravity that governs the flow of water.

It is the same for your health. You were designed to heal! The only reason you are still sick is there are obstacles or barriers to your innate healing ability. I have been a doctor for nearly forty years. I have never healed anyone. My job is to find the obstacles and facilitate their removal and your body does the rest. It is a beautiful thing!

Understanding barriers and obstacles will help you understand why taking good supplements for your thyroid didn't work, or didn't work as well as they could have. If you have inflammation, you have to put out the fires before you can rebuild.

Beth was smart and had done a ton of reading online about natural solutions for her thyroid. She brought in supplement bottles to show me. A thyroid formula from a good company that I respect and even some selenium. She had learned that this mineral is needed to convert T4 into T3, the active form of thyroid hormone. She couldn't understand why they weren't working until we talked about putting out the fires of inflammation first, then rebuilding.

Here are the 5 steps to healing your thyroid;
1. Prepare and support
2. Kill the bad bugs/hidden infections
3. Restore and replenish the gut
4. Rebalance hormones
5. Detox

Step One is often overlooked in the healing process. Doing so puts the cart before the horse. We need to move toxic wastes out of the body in order to reduce inflammation and to do so requires that we prepare the body and support your elimination channels. We are talking about the liver and kidneys, the main organs of elimination. In Step Two we will attack the hidden infections. This produces a lot of metabolic debris and toxic cellular bits and pieces. If we miss step one, these wastes have no easy way out and so they recirculate and make you feel terrible.

Eliminating metabolic waste occurs in phases. If all the phases are not working, the wastes back up. Think of this process as taking out the garbage from the kitchen. Phase one gets it to the back door. Phase two gets it outside to the trash can. What if phase two isn't working well? The trash stacks up by the back door and pretty soon the whole house smells. This is why Step One is so important. Your body needs to be able to take the trash out all the way. This is also why being constipated makes you feel so awful. You are not able to eliminate wastes and some of the toxins get reabsorbed back into your body.

Step Two is about putting out the fires of inflammation by attacking any hidden infections. If you have a chronic health problem, I can almost guarantee you have one or more low grade infections. This includes one or more of these microbes: bacteria, viruses, mold and parasites. These infections drive an inflammatory response. We help your immune system do its job of killing these invaders. When microorganisms die, they leave behind metabolic waste and debris. This is why, when you have an acute infection like a cold, you feel so awful. The waste from these dead bugs is toxic.

Step Three is repairing and replenishing your gut. We refer to the microorganisms living in your gut, especially the large intestine, as the microbiome. Your microbiome helps boost your immune system, interacts with your central nervous system and affects brain chemistry, protects you from toxins entering your bloodstream, helps you digest your food and absorb nutrients, helps control blood pressure, makes B vitamins and vitamin K and so much more. In a healthy person almost all the bacteria living there are beneficial. In chronic illness the ratio of bad bugs to good bugs gets lopsided. Step Two is about killing off the bad ones. Now we restore a healthy balance. There are about ten trillion cells in your body. There are about 100 trillion microbes living in your gut. They outnumber us ten to one and we literally can't live without them. Think of your gut as a hotel with 100 trillion rooms. In chronic illness the hotel is run down and a bunch of gang members have moved in. In Step Two we evict those bad elements and in Step Three we restore your hotel to a 5-star accommodation so we can invite our VIP guests, the healthy bacteria, to live and thrive.

Step Four is balancing hormones. You might be asking yourself why we didn't begin with this step . Hypothyroid is about not having enough thyroid hormone to keep your body energized and functioning like it should, so why not just give the body what it is lacking? The answer is that your cells have to be ready to receive and respond to the hormone messages. They can't do that properly when they are inflamed. Imagine trying to fill up your car with gasoline without opening the gas cap. Pouring gasoline all over your car is not going to make it run. Your cells need to be able to receive the hormone signals. For most patients, they can really feel themselves turning the corner to big improvements in energy and a significant reduction in their other symptoms at this point. You can feel the healing taking place. Improvements have been happening along the way with the first three steps but now it is more obvious.

Step Five is detox. Many think of this as a deep liver cleanse or a gallbladder flush. It needs to go much further. The toxins in your body are not just confined to the liver and gallbladder. They are potentially in every cell. This is why detox needs to happen on a cellular level and must include detoxing the brain itself. Beth was apprehensive when we talked about this as her next step. She told me about a friend who had done a liver detox and a gallbladder flush and ended up in the emergency room with horrible abdominal pains and feeling like she had been beaten by a club. Again, this is because things were done in the wrong order. You must have your detoxification pathways and channels open before attempting a deep cellular level detox. This means the liver and bowel must be working properly BEFORE you try moving massive amounts of cellular level toxins out of the body. Done correctly, you should not even feel you are detoxing. The process should be smooth and in the background.

We are exposed to tens of thousands of chemicals. Most of which have not been tested for safety. Heavy metals lurk in underarm deodorants, lipstick, mercury amalgam dental fillings, flu shots and other vaccinations. Glyphosate, PCBs, any number of pesticides and herbicides are out there. No matter how careful you are in limiting your exposure you can't escape them all. And why is it important to eliminate toxins? Because they drive…say it with me…inflammation! And inflammation is the root driver of all degenerative disease.

Now that you understand a bit more about the five steps you might say this would be a good approach to any degenerative disease or health concern. You would be right. When you work on repairing and healing the body on a cellular level, good things happen. This is your roadmap to sustained improved quality of life and sidestepping other diseases that you would invite in by not knowing and following this strategy.

Thyroid Friendly Lifestyle

Diet, sleep, fasting, drinking enough water, sensible exercise, stress management. There is more we could add here but these lifestyle measures go a long way.

If you have an autoimmune disease, you should eliminate gluten from your diet.

Sleep is when you heal. Not enough quality/quantity of sleep and you are always playing catch up and hindering your ability to heal.

Fasting could be a book by itself and there are some good ones out there. I will just say that if I were on the proverbial desert island

and could only pick one recommendation for lifestyle, I would pick fasting. It is that powerful.

Most of us need to drink more water. A good target is half your body weight in ounces.

Keep exercise simple. For most patients, I like variable resistance exercise done every other day and walking on the off day.

Stress is part of the human condition. We all have it. Don't stress about having stress! Exercise, music, meditation, spirituality, nature, puttering in the garden. Find what works for you.

If you have or suspect hypothyroid, it is likely not your thyroid's fault. You probably have an autoimmune condition for which there is no medical cure. Now you know the rest of the story. You were born to heal. Let's find the barriers that are in your body's way, remove them through functional nutrition and stand back and watch the magic happen as you get your life back.

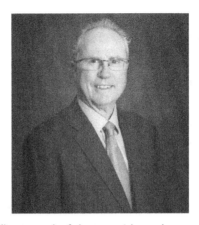

For over thirty-five wonderful years, I have been serving my local community as a doctor of chiropractic, striving to help people like you achieve their optimal health. I graduated with honors from the prestigious Life West College of Chiropractic and, since then, I've been on a lifelong journey of learning, and regularly attend seminars to stay on the cutting edge within my field. I was born and raised in the Bay Area of California and completed my undergraduate degree in Chemistry from Brigham Young University in 1981. After graduating from chiropractic school, I chose to bring up my family in the beautiful small town of Cody, WY, where I've had the privilege of helping many thousands of individuals enjoy a more vibrant life.

My passion has always been to identify the root cause of problems and to correct physiological dysfunction, which has since then brought better living to thousands of patients. With over 35 years of experience in treating spine-related complaints and my advanced training in functional medicine, spinal decompression, posture correction, neurological rehabilitation, extremities, laser therapy, and clinical nutrition, I am well equipped to handle challenging cases.

I enjoy snowboarding, backpacking, fly fishing, and most of all, being a grandpa. My intention with this book is to welcome you into our ProHealth family and help you embark on your personal journey to a healthier, happier life.

https://www.prohealthwyoming.com/ | drshane@prohealthwyoming.com

CHAPTER 7:

Healing the Body to Heal the Brain

By: Sandy Wesson BSN, RN, FNTP, CGP

The Gut-Brain Connection

Rachel was experiencing life as an active nineteen-year-old until she was hit by a drunk driver. Though she had struggled with digestive issues, anxiety, and depression prior to the accident, at that moment, this young woman who enjoyed horseback riding and other activities was changed to a person who experienced confusion, uncertainty, more profound anxiety, depression, and was on medication to help with these symptoms. This was a nightmare for both Rachel and her family. Fortunately, her mom Barb is a strong advocate who kept searching for help.

To help you, the reader, understand her story and more importantly, to understand that there is hope, Rachel described her experience:

"I experienced drastic mood changes, really high highs and really low lows. I had a lot of rage. I had all the symptoms of TBI (traumatic brain injury). I was diagnosed with IBS (irritable bowel syndrome) as I had a really unhappy stomach. It was constantly hurting. Most

foods hurt my tummy, and I was very irregular. Two things that I noticed drastically changed once I started my supplement program, my mood was more stable, and my gut was much happier. I had done neurofeedback for six years before meeting Sandy. It worked great initially, but I didn't seem to make much more progress with it after a few years. That became frustrating and a little scary as I had completely relied on it to keep me stable. I can now confidently say that I have never been more confident without it"!

At the time of this writing, with the help of her doctor, Rachel is weaning off the medications she has been taking for anxiety and depression.

This is from Barb, Rachel's mom:

"Our saga began almost nine years ago, when my nineteen-year-old daughter Rachel's car was hit by a drunk driver. I was called to the hospital, where no attention was paid to the swelling on her forehead. I began to realize there was something very wrong when she couldn't walk straight, was dizzy and nauseous, and both pupils were hugely dilated. Then began a string of various professionals, some helpful, some not. I was told that we are in primitive times regarding brain injury, and I found that to be very evident when trying to find help. We spent eight years working on helping her recover before we found Sandy.

Apparently, many professionals do not know that Traumatic Brain Injury can affect every cell in your body and digestion dysfunction is very common.

Once we found Sandy at Brainworks For Life, life improved! We went straight to work on digestion, and Sandy was able to convince my daughter to actually take the supplements she recommended and follow the plan Sandy devised.

Sandy is a warm, caring, knowledgeable person who gives her all. She is really helping us, and I firmly believe she can help you too!"

In Rachel's own words, "my life has significantly improved since we began with Sandy. Being able to digest food properly has given me the freedom and confidence I never thought I would have again. My emotions are more normal, and I'm not desperately changing medications all the time to try to find relief. I notice a huge difference when I do not follow my program. Sandy has helped me in many ways, supporting and mentoring me through this journey. My body has healed in many ways I did not think possible." We both highly recommend Sandy and Brainworks For Life.

Barb

The education I provided to Rachel and her mom, Barb, is similar to the information I am providing to you.

If you want the short version—medical doctors are not taught about digestion and the effects that bad digestion has on our body and our brain. Concussions make everything worse. Our digestion must be healed to heal our brain.

If you want a detailed version of how and why this happens, read on.

Life / Health is dependent on our cellular function. Where does our energy come from? Inside our cells are mitochondria, which make energy. These mitochondria are our "energizer bunnies". Every cell of our body has 1000 mitochondria per cell. The liver and the heart have about 5000 mitochondria per cell. The brain has 10,000 mitochondria *per* cell. Our brain needs a lot of energy to function well!

It is worth mentioning that our mitochondria have more than one job. If we are fighting an infection for example, mitochondria have a role in our immune system. They call in the killer cells to fight the battle. They can't easily do more than one job, so if they are helping the body fight an infection, they can't make as much energy. In this scenario, where will we notice it first? Since the brain has 10,000 mitochondria per cell, requiring a LOT of energy, we may notice brain fog or brain fatigue before we have full-on physical symptoms. This is an oversimplified explanation, but...... you get the picture.

If we are not digesting our food, if we are not breaking down our food and *absorbing* nutrition, we are not getting nutrition to the cells which means we are not getting nutrition to the mitochondria where energy is made.

People often ask me about the gut-brain connection. What is it? How are the gut and brain connected? Let's break it down. A significant connection between the gut and the brain is the vagus nerve, which is the longest nerve in the body. The vagus nerve starts in the brain, it connects to the heart and the lungs, and ends in the gut. This is important to understand because the gut has its own communication system, known as the enteric nervous system. Approximately 100 million nerve cells are in the human intestine. That roughly equals the number of nerve cells in the spinal cord. You may have heard the saying that "the gut is the second brain". This is an important part of our body's communication system.

To understand the gut-brain connection, we first need to understand the gut. The function of our gut affects cellular health and immune health. It affects our mental health, and it affects our brain health. I am talking about digestion—how well we break down food, and how well we absorb the food we eat.

Digestion is a complex process with many things that can cause problems, so I will try to simplify the explanation but also give you enough information to understand the process. Hang in there with me.

Ideally, we should be able to enjoy a meal and digest it easily. Poor digestion may result in burping, gas, acid reflux, diarrhea, or constipation.

What are things that impact digestion? Well, breaking down our food starts with chewing. Each bite should be chewed about thirty times (yes, really!), resulting in the food being almost liquid when we swallow. This is important because amylase, an enzyme that breaks down carbohydrates, is only provided in the mouth from the salivary gland. If we gulp our food without adequate chewing, the food goes to the stomach without breakdown by amylase. Digestion is now behind the game. The digestive juices in the stomach are trying to break down food particles which are larger than they should be. When conditions are right – when the stomach is at the proper pH—the partially digested food is moved to the small intestine. If conditions are not right to be moved to the small intestine, it stays in the stomach and ferments and putrefies. This causes gas (bubbles). Putrefied food can also move back up the esophagus and cause heartburn. This is acid reflux, also known as GERD, Gastroesophageal Reflux Disease. The solution to GERD is **NOT** taking prescription medication to decrease the acid in your stomach. The solution is to fix the problem in the first place. You may need more digestive enzymes or hydrochloric acid (Hcl), which breaks down proteins. This means you may need *more* acid to digest food. There are a variety of reasons your body may not be making adequate amounts of enzymes and Hcl. I won't go into these reasons in this writing.

From the stomach the partially or fully digested food moves to the first portion of the small intestine, which is where we absorb our nutrients. There are little finger-like villi with tiny, microscopic holes. The liquified food surrounds those little villi and moves through the microscopic holes to absorb nutrients. What happens if we didn't chew our food well enough or if we don't have enough enzymes or hydrochloric acid to digest? If the food hasn't been digested well, there are large pieces such as proteins that are trying to get through the microscopic holes. They won't fit, so these pieces start pushing through the cells that make the intestinal lining, through what is known as the tight junction of the small intestine. When these protein molecules start making holes in the intestinal wall and pushing through—now we've got leaky gut.

A leaky gut allows not only undigested food particles into the bloodstream, but other toxins as well. What happens now? Our immune system, which is (or should be) always paying attention, sees these particles as "foreign invaders." As the immune system starts doing its job of attacking foreign invaders, in time it can get confused and start attacking our own cells/tissues. This is known as autoimmune. Autoimmune issues can appear in different places in our bodies, such as rheumatoid arthritis, systemic lupus erythematosus, multiple sclerosis, Hashimoto's thyroiditis and more. In the bowels, inflammatory bowel disease (IBD) can develop. The immune system attacks the lining of the intestines, causing episodes of diarrhea, rectal bleeding, urgent bowel movements, abdominal pain, fever and weight loss. Ulcerative colitis and Crohn's disease are the two major forms of IBD.

How does IBD and poor gut health affect the brain? In oh so many ways. It has been known by scientists for some time that the gut and brain communicate with each other via the vagus nerve. A newer understanding is that the gut microbiota (the microscopic organisms of a particular environment) also works within this communication. This connection makes up the microbiota-gut-brain axis.

The gut contains several different microorganisms that are mostly bacteria but also include fungi and viruses. These microbes are a microbiota, also known as the microbiome.

The body and the gut microbiota can live in a beneficial relationship. While in the colon, they feed on fiber and other remnants of digestion. As a result, they can support the health of the brain and body.

The brain gets a lot of information from the gut, but the brain also sends some messages to the digestive tract. For example, the brain-to-gut messages sent via the vagus nerve control the release of stomach acid and digestive enzymes. For example, the very thought of eating can release the stomach's juices before food gets there. They also impact inflammation levels, and how the body responds to stress.

The messages the vagus nerve carries are heavily influenced by microbiota. When microbes release neurotransmitters such as serotonin and dopamine, these can switch on the vagus nerve for transmission to the brain. Serotonin is known as the "feel good" neurotransmitter. Eighty percent of our serotonin is made in the gut and is dependent on a sufficient number of good bacteria.

When the microbiota is diverse and includes more beneficial, or "good" microbes, the body will have better communication, or "messaging." But when the gut bacteria are out of balance (more bad bacteria than beneficial bacteria), the communication changes. In this case, people are more likely to develop gut problems, brain issues and mental health issues such as anxiety and depression.

What about the Brain-Gut Connection? How can trauma to the brain affect digestion?

Meet Chris.

Nearly a year ago I got into a bad car accident that left me with a severe brain injury and whiplash! I had all the symptoms of a Traumatic Brain injury. After seeking help from multiple practices and physicians, six months later I still was not able to function normally from day to day. I certainly couldn't work in my field of construction! I was at a loss of what to do until I got referred to BrainWorks!

The treatment I received at Brainworks was a life saver. Their approach to treating brain injuries, I believe, is crucial to a good recovery. I did both nutrition and Neurofeedback.

As someone who has struggled with dietary problems for years, only after my accident and coming to BrainWorks, did I realize how much our gut affects our brain and inflammation! After treating my gut, they were then able to help heal my brain with the Neurofeedback therapy. I am now able to fully function from day to day and my progression with my recovery is drastic and, unlike the other treatments I did before BrainWorks, it is permanent!

Thank You so much to the lovely ladies at BrainWorks! I will be forever appreciative of your help!"

Chris already had issues with digestion when he was in a car accident resulting in brain trauma. The brain trauma made the digestion worse, which did not allow his brain to heal. "Leaky gut, leaky brain".

What if someone has **good digestion-no** gut issues, then experiences a concussion? For ninety-five percent of people, their digestion will be negatively impacted within three days. Why does this happen? Let's go back to the vagus nerve. Remember, it starts in the brain and ends in the digestive tract, which has its own nervous system – the enteric nervous system. When a head injury occurs, there is a trauma to the brain resulting in inflammation. This "shock" travels down the vagus nerve and now brings the "shock" to the enteric nervous system, creating inflammation in the gut. Now we have a case of "leaky brain causing leaky gut, which keeps the gut inflamed, causing leaky brain. At a time when we need to have intact tight junctions (intact cellular barriers) in both the gut and the Blood Brain Barrier (BBB), both are leaky, so neither can heal. Both the gut and the brain remain inflamed, as happened to the clients introduced above. This cycle of leaky gut, leaky brain can go on for years. The brain has a capacity to heal, but only when we break the cycle of inflammation.

When working with someone who has a new concussion, I have a protocol to get the inflammation down in the brain quickly and prevent digestion issues, though if digestion issues have already developed, quickly support the gut to heal. It is better to prevent the longstanding issues of the brain and gut, but as you have seen with Rachel and Chris, we can still affect the gut and brain months and years later.

Common Causes of Inflammation

Gut: food sensitivities such as gluten, dairy, soy, sugar, environmental toxins such as herbicides, pesticides, glyphosate, mold, parasites, many chemicals, concussions.

Brain: food sensitivities such as gluten, dairy, soy, sugar, environmental toxins such as herbicides, pesticides, glyphosate, mold, parasites, radiation, concussions, heavy metals such as mercury, lead and aluminum.

Infections: in our teeth and chronic sinus infections can also travel to our brain. Lyme— Borellia and co-infections of Bartonella and Babesia can also infect the brain causing neurological symptoms. Epstein- Barr Virus (mononucleosis) is a virus which can cause neurological inflammation. It is important to address the infections themselves, but also support gut and brain health.

Mold: Mold is very commonly overlooked, so I want to explain why it is important to make sure it is not part of the picture of poor health. Those who carry a specific gene called the HLA-DR gene, can have difficulty recovering from mold and other toxin exposures. Thus, for twenty-five percent of people, mold is a significant hurdle to regaining health.

When living or working in a building with mold (most of the time we have no idea there is mold) we breathe in the mycotoxins and possibly the mold spores themselves. Mold can affect our brain as well as our gut, resulting in gut-brain dysfunction. Mold has a significant negative effect on the mitochondria (our energy batteries). Remember I said earlier that brain cells have 10,000 mitochondria per cell, so if mold is making it difficult for the mitochondria to make energy, decreased function will happen throughout the body, but especially the brain.

Thoughts, Traumas and Toxins

An army veteran came to me for help with anxiety and depression as well as PTSD and multiple concussions. He had served two tours in Afghanistan. The VA doctors wanted to give him antidepressants. Thankfully, this man wanted to "get better, not just mask the symptoms." He had heard about the use of neurofeedback to address anxiety and depression and to treat concussions.

As I began to evaluate my client, it became clear that he had extreme inflammation in both his gut and his brain. In addition to multiple concussions, he had been exposed to *many* toxins as well as parasites, while serving. Prior to deployment, he had lived in moldy barracks, and received many vaccines in a short period of time, which is harder on the immune system than when given spread out over time. In Afghanistan the exposure to multiple toxins was very high.

I explained that while neurofeedback can be helpful to heal the brain, it would be a better use of his money to first take him through a cellular detox to clean up his body and brain. We discussed the role of mitochondria and the need to improve mitochondrial function for his body and brain to regain health. In his case this meant healing digestion and clearing the many toxins from his body as a starting point.

Neurofeedback. Since I have mentioned neurofeedback a few times, let me explain neurofeedback, then we will come back to the story of my client.

Trauma to the brain (whether emotional, physical or toxins) can affect your brain's function. Brainwaves can get stuck in abnormal patterns, which can cause issues such as low power / brain fog, anxiety, depression, issues with memory, motivation, anger, and more.

Neurofeedback is a technology which utilizes the brain's ability to change itself (neuroplasticity) to bring about improvement in brain function. As described above, symptoms such as brain fog, anxiety, depression, issues with memory, motivation, anger, and other symptoms can interfere with the enjoyment we experience. This approach trains the brain to function optimally, thus improving attention, mood, learning ability and more without the use of medication.

How Does Neurofeedback Work?

Neurofeedback works by helping patients retrain their brain activity, which is measured as brainwaves.

There are four primary types of brainwaves that serve different purposes in the brain. While they are all necessary for proper functioning, disruptions can occur when one brainwave becomes dominant at the wrong time, resulting in poor cognitive functioning, stress, anxiety, and more.

Below is a breakdown of the 4 primary types of brainwaves and when they occur:

1. Beta Waves

Beta waves are the highest (i.e., fastest) frequency waves. They occur when the brain is actively engaged in a task, like taking an exam, giving a presentation, solving a problem, or having a conversation. You'll feel alert and "at the ready" when these waves are dominant.

1. Alpha Waves

These are the next fastest frequency brainwaves. They are present when the brain is in a more relaxed state and can make you feel satisfied or at ease. When you close your eyes to relax or meditate, your brain produces more alpha brainwaves.

1. Theta Waves

Slower than alpha waves, theta brain waves are present when we are sleepy or daydreaming. These waves help us get ready to "shut down" at the end of the day. They can also disrupt our thought patterns if they occur at the wrong time—like when you're studying for a test or in a meeting with your boss. Excess theta waves are frequently the cause of poor focus and attention, as is often the case with individuals with ADD/ADHD.

1. Delta Waves

The slowest frequency brainwave, delta waves, become predominant primarily when we are in a state of deep, dreamless sleep.

Brains that produce too many slow-frequency waves and not enough high-frequency waves (or vice versa) won't function at an optimal level.

If your brain is stuck in an unhealthy functioning pattern, you may feel an overwhelming sense of fatigue or like you're living in a fog or feel agitation or restlessness.

Moreover, it may become difficult to focus on even the easiest tasks, which can seriously reduce your quality of life.

During a neurofeedback session, sensors are placed on your scalp. These sensors measure electrical activity in the brain and generate an electroencephalogram (EEG).

Your brain will interact with computer software, based on your brainwave activity. The signals sent back to the brain create a change in your brainwaves.

This disrupts the brain that is "stuck" in certain ways of functioning and allows the brain to reorganize in more optimal ways of functioning. Like when you reboot your frozen computer, neurofeedback can help get you out of unhealthy brain patterns.

OK, let's return to the story of the Veteran with brain trauma, PTSD, and *many* toxins. As I stated earlier, this man came seeking healing, not to have his symptoms covered up. I applaud this client. Our veterans deserve more than a Band-Aid.

In addition to having him fill out a questionnaire of symptoms and doing a physical exam to evaluate inflammation in his gut, I also did a QEEG evaluation of his brain function. After reviewing all the data, I explained that for his brain to heal, we must address the toxins in his body and brain, and we need to heal his gut.

We agreed to start stabilizing his messed-up gut, starting to work on digestion. Just with this beginning point he began to pass parasites in his bowel movements. This usually happens when we start giving herbal products to kill parasites. To have it happen when just working on digestion was an indication that parasites were a big problem, and they were having a strong negative effect on his health.

Parasites eat the nutrients meant for us, and their poop is detrimental to us. In addition, just as our bodies create neurotransmitters which influence the way we feel, parasites also create their own neurotransmitters, which impact us. Parasites don't just stay in the digestive tract. They can move into the pancreas, liver, gallbladder, lungs, brain, and other areas of the body. I won't go into detail about eliminating parasites, however, it is important to understand that parasites are way more common than we are led to believe. Many clients improve physical and mental health when we address parasites.

Over the months, as we moved through the phases of cellular detox (removing toxins from the cells so that mitochondria can do their job) I wanted to assess the effects on his brain. At no cost to him, I did a QEEG brain map before we started each new phase of detox. This is not something I routinely do, but this man had so many concussions and was so toxic, I wanted to see what kind of changes were occurring.

The first few months the brain showed minor changes, but the changes became more pronounced in months three and four. The changes I saw on the brain maps correlated with the improvements he was experiencing with decreased anxiety and depression. In addition to using herbal products to kill parasites and remove chemicals, we continued to support digestion and mitochondrial function. At months seven and eight, as we were removing heavy metals from his body and brain, he stated that he was making better decisions and not having the anger issues he had been experiencing prior. PTSD can bring up anger issues, but there is also an area of the brain that regulates emotion, including anger. With a traumatic brain injury, damage to that area can cause anger and rage in a person who did not experience these emotions prior to the injury. This can cause confusion and feelings of guilt for some, as I have seen in other clients. In addition to detoxing his body, this veteran worked with a mental health therapist for a few months to help manage PTSD.

This is an example of how the brain can heal when we remove the toxins and address infections in the body and brain. If you, or someone you know has had a concussion, even a minor one, do a check-in with yourself. How is your digestion? How is your emotional status? Focus and memory? If any of this is off, get help if needed, but start working on healing your gut TODAY.

How do I assess the needs of my clients?

I read the bloodwork you already have from your doctor, but I read it from a functional perspective, which gives me so much important information.

I want to be aware of all your symptoms, so you will complete a questionnaire of symptoms.

I do muscle testing—working with your body's innate wisdom. This helps to identify the supplements *your* body needs. No guessing.

If we are considering neurofeedback, we will do a brain map evaluation of brain waves.

Tips and Tools to help your brain work for life:

Eat nutrient dense whole food, preferably organic.

Avoid processed foods.

Early morning hydration. First thing in the morning, before you drink coffee or anything else, drink a glass of clean filtered water. Add some electrolytes to the water for even better results. During the night, our brain shrinks slightly while it is doing its process of detox. This glass of water will wake up our brain as well as wake up our digestive tract.

Exercise—movement helps keep oxygenated blood flowing to your brain.

Community: engage with family and friends.

Regular sleep.

Healthy digestion.

Neurofeedback to assist brainwaves to return to optimal function.

Nutrients for the Brain: These are a few basic nutrients. There are many others.

Omega 3s—healthy fats. Our cell walls are made primarily of fat.

B vitamins—a deficiency of B vitamins has been shown to increase anxiety and depression. If you have methylation issues, it is important to take methylated B.

Magnesium

Clean, filtered water

Help for digestion:

Chew your food well.

Supplement with digestive enzymes and Hcl if you are deficient.

Avoid foods you are sensitive to.

Avoid gluten- Wheat and many other grains are treated with glyphosate, which causes leaky gut and is known to cause some types of cancer.

Increase fiber in your diet.

Probiotics, including fermented foods which act as a probiotic.

The Pulse Test: developed by Arthur F. Coca, MD. This test will help you know if a particular food may be an issue for you. It is also known as the Coca Pulse Test.

Test Procedure

1. Wait at least two hours after you have eaten.
2. You need to relax for a few minutes before starting the test and throughout the test.

3. Take your pulse for a full 60 seconds. We need a full minute because we don't want any rounding errors. (Do not take it for 15 seconds and multiply by 4, or 30 seconds x 2).
4. Put a piece of food in your mouth. Chew it for 30 seconds to 1 minute, but do not swallow any of it.
5. Take your pulse again, for a full minute, with the food in your mouth but without swallowing it.
6. Spit out the food. Rinse out your mouth with water and spit out the rinse.
7. Let your pulse return to your baseline before testing another food. Then repeat.

If your pulse increased by six beats or more, you had a stress reaction to that food. Avoid it for at least a month, and then test it again.

My Journey

I was recently asked how/why I chose brain and gut health as a focus. As is frequently the case for practitioners, it chose me. I was living a life of health challenges which I did not understand. Working as a nurse I experienced digestion issues, fatigue, muscle aches and brain fog for many years. Looking back…… was it from being bitten in my twenties, the bite resulting in a big bullseye rash which I now know can indicate Lyme and co-infections? Was it from being scratched by a monkey in South Africa while celebrating my 25th wedding anniversary? (It was a deep, dirty wound. The monkey was after the food in my hand.) Was it from unknowingly living in mold for many years? Was it from concussions? Was it from being exposed to many infections during my years as a nurse? Was it from stress? Or did all of these things result in my bucket becoming full to overflowing so that my body could no longer carry this toxic load?

After working as a nurse for many years, my healing began when I went back to school and became a Functional Nutritional Therapy Practitioner, which gave me a deep understanding of digestion, digestion dysfunction and the effects on the body. I then began studying cellular detoxification with dedicated, knowledgeable mentors. This was critical to my own healing, and I have found cellular detox to be important for many of my clients as well.

I do believe that our bodies can heal, with help. That help may be in the form of releasing old belief patterns, addressing head injuries, cleaning up our diets and giving the cells the nutrition needed to function, and cleaning out the toxins we have been exposed to.

Thoughts. Traumas. Toxins. My hope is that every one of you will dig a little deeper into your own health issues, get the help you need to renew your health and enjoy life!

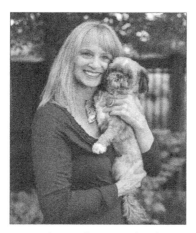

Sandy has been a Registered Nurse for forty-two years, and a Functional Nutritional Therapy Practitioner for eight years. Her work as an RN includes several years in the Intensive Care Unit as well as end-of-life care as a Palliative Care and Hospice Nurse. She now owns her own business helping people regain health through nutrition, detoxification, addressing issues with digestion and brain dysfunction. Neurofeedback is a tool she uses to help brain function.

Sandy enjoys being in nature, playing with her dog Tara, and spending time with her large extended family. She experiences joy when she sees her clients regain health and begin to enjoy life again!

Sandy Wesson BSN, RN, FNTP, CGP

Detoxification Specialist

Functional Bloodwork Specialist

Neurofeedback Provider

Ph: 541.639.8400

BrainWorksforLife@gmail.com

www.brainworksforlife.com

Facebook: www.facebook.com/BrainWorksForLife

Instagram: www.instagram.com/brainworks_for_life

CHAPTER 8:

Wellness to Weight Loss

By: Dr. Angela Rahm B.C.N.D.

Y ou get healthy to lose weight, not lose weight to get healthy!

How Did I Get Here? That's the question I asked myself when I was forty-six and on vacation. As I was getting dressed, I leaned into the bathroom mirror, shook my head and looked up and said, «what has happened to me?" Even as I write this, tears fill my eyes, as if it were yesterday, and the memory of that time in my life is like salt in a new wound. This particular night was the turning point in my life. After three trips in two and half months, it was easier to wash and repack the same clothes because I knew they were the clothes that fit me on the first trip which were already my "fat" clothes…You can see where this is going and you are right. The third trip was the straw that broke the camel's back. It wasn't that they were tight, they completely did not fit! So, I had to attend a large and influential social event on that last trip with unbuttoned slacks!

Having survived that night, and that trip, I came back a different woman. I did what any normal, desperate, but motivated woman would do and I hired a trainer and went on ANOTHER DIET! What I realized though, was that you can't out-train a bad and inconsistent diet. I could not have four good diet days and three party-like-a-Rockstar days, repeat each and every week, and expect quick and life changing results!

Like many, I have spent the vast majority of my life on, or thinking about, a DIET. From the early age of eleven into my fifties I had been focused on losing weight. I finally came to the realization that all diets can fail, and all diets can work, and that it's not just about the D.I.E.T (Did I Eat That). In this chapter, my promise is to give you solid foundational tips and steps to get results, leaving you with more energy, ability to lose excess weight and loving the body you are in once again.

Finally, the realization I had to fully accept, was that my lifestyle habits were not 100% aligned with the result I envisioned for myself and I had no one or nothing else to blame. I had a crazy busy life, like everyone. I worked hard, played hard, and tried to be and do everything for everyone. Life was good and life was exhausting. I had no balance and no time which led me to poor choices, creating unhealthy habits, depressed, frustrated and 35lbs.+ overweight.

It was also in this phase of my life that my son was suffering from an undiagnosed illness, later to be determined to be Chronic Lyme Disease, and my best friend with Cancer for the second time. Things got real, real fast, and I became extremely passionate about natural health. Shortly after this, I made the decision to sell my franchise businesses, went back to school, and became a Board-Certified Naturopathic Doctor.

If you are thinking to yourself, "I've been there," or maybe you are there right now, my desire is to give you HOPE that there is a way to get YOU back!

You, like many, may need a program that is designed specifically for you. I too have hired many professionals, paid thousands for programs and courses, read hundreds of books, and listened to countless podcasts to learn as much as I could to help myself, my family and friends, and my patients, to figure out the best approaches for optimal health and "sustainable" weight loss. This constant cycle is what prompted the creation of the Wellness to Weight Loss program.

When it comes to diet for weight loss, remember, any diet can work and any diet can fail. Sometimes your lab findings alone can wake you up and have your mindset shifted to take your health more seriously. The event style dieters, you know, the ones that want to lose 10-15lbs. for a wedding, vacation, reunion… they never keep the weight off and will usually continue yo-yo dieting, doing more harm than good. No matter how much weight you think you have to lose, it is important to understand that fad diets (like keto), medications (like Ozempic) and extreme exercises (like Crossfit) are not a good fit for most, especially if you are menopausal, stressed, and have underlying health issues.

I understand in some cases these things work, but it's usually not sustainable for most. Even those who have tried extreme methods often find themselves bigger, injured, more tired and feeling even worse, because another "thing" didn't work!

When you are trying to incorporate a healthier diet and relieve some of the internal stress, what is important is to focus on whole foods. I know, easy right? If it were that easy no one would be overweight and I would not be writing this chapter. Obviously, there is a process in eating the right food, in the right portions, at the right times, and in the right combinations, that will fast track your maintainable weight loss and healthier lifestyle.

Our patients focus on a variety of protein, 2-3 servings a day. The majority of people are not getting a sufficient amount of protein, which are the building blocks that support a healthy musculoskeletal system and maintain muscle integrity.

Healthy fats are important for the brain, joints, gut, liver, and every cell in the body. Good choices would be, olive and coconut oils, ghee, organic butter, avocados, macadamia nuts, walnuts and pecans. Keep in mind eggs and animal proteins also have a good amount of fats.

Carbohydrates are a hot topic. How much, what kind, how often? It is crazy how many "theories" there are around carbs. We recommend our patients focus on non-starchy vegetables, avoiding things like corn, peas, and white potatoes. We have them choose lower glycemic foods by limiting grains, legumes, dairy and sugar (stevia is one exception because it is an herb and is not a big insulin-glucose trigger for most) for at least six weeks. We then have a structured food reintroduction process to help bring back foods the individual can't see themselves living without.

It's important to pay attention to how you feel during this process as food sensitivities could cause bloating, gas, fatigue, headaches, or weight gain.

Fruits are often demonized because of the sugar content. Most people love fruit, but let's be clear, it is fructose, which is a form of sugar, so it must be treated as such. We suggest choosing lower glycemic fruits like berries. This does not mean you can't enjoy a chunk of pineapple or watermelon slab now and then, but we do not recommend eating too much in one sitting or in one day. The human body is one big puzzle and the diet should always be the first step in the process for addressing any struggles you may be dealing with.

Now that we have established basic dietary recommendations let's discuss Intermittent Fasting (IF). IF is not another fad diet and in fact, it has been scientifically and clinically proven to be very effective for overall wellness and weight loss. Many over-think this and believe there's no way to limit their eating window and fear they'll go into starvation mode. There are also many who are stuck in the old belief system that everyone should eat three meals and two to three snacks per day which in most cases actually spikes glucose and insulin all day long forcing the body to store this excess in the fat cells. Focus on two solid meals per day and if needed, then have a protein snack to help power through your day.

For optimal health, one should actually not eat three hours before bed or within the first two hours of waking up. This constitutes a base level of intermittent fasting. IF allows a flexible eating window around individual lifestyles, i.e., work/career, current health status, any habits needed to be broken, to become a successful way of life. There are too many studies to support the benefits of IF to not have this as a key foundation.

Pro tip: If new to the IF concept, consider starting with a twelve hour fast. During this time frame you can consume water, tea and black coffee. Keep in mind, seven to eight hours of this fasting period is generally spent sleeping. There are a lot of benefits to working your way up to an extended fasting window. However, if you have underlying health issues we recommend always consulting with a qualified health professional.

If you have your diet in check, and you're still struggling, it could be due to hormonal imbalances. The body needs cholesterol to make sex hormones like Progesterone, Cortisol, DHEA, Testosterone and Estrogen. Diet, stress, medications and genetic factors could be hindering your ability to make and balance these hormones. This is another reason we test ..... and do not guess. In the traditional medical establishment, testing is often inaccurate and is used to medicate or give justification to perform surgeries rather than treating the cause of hormonal imbalances. There are circumstances that medications and the use of bio-identical hormone replacement therapy may be beneficial. We take a holistic approach with our patients and address each one individually as we believe lifestyle choices, diet and supplementation are the key foundations for optimal hormonal health.

Another misunderstood hormone is Insulin. Insulin and blood sugar are very important to lose weight and keep it off. Insulin is a fat storing hormone and if the body loses its ability to recognize it, it can't carry the glucose into the cell to be converted into energy. If this process fails, the energy (glucose) will get stored in your fat cells. The frequent reoccurrence of this process could lead you to become insulin resistant.

Symptoms you may experience are obesity, increased subcutaneous fat around the midsection, increased appetite and cravings, poor sleep, high triglycerides, higher than normal blood pressure, arteriosclerosis, slow wound healing, PCOS (polycystic ovarian syndrome), high liver markers, poor memory, thinning hair, chronic infections like bacterial and fungal low-grade infections, gum disorders, skin problems, skin tags, and excess thirst. Insulin resistance is a precursor to diabetes and getting blood sugar under control is very important. Blood sugar signals insulin to be released from the pancreas. If there is too much glucose and you are insulin resistant it will not be able to convert to energy and will be stored in your fat cells. Once again, this can quickly be reversed with proper diet. We have patients who have been on insulin for over twenty years whose medical doctors convinced them they will be for the rest of their lives, only to work with us and have their physician take them off within six weeks.

When it comes to the inability to lose weight, feeling fatigued and brain fog, and having your hair fall out, we are quick to go to our medical professionals and get our thyroid tested. The standard of care in the medical community for thyroid testing is TSH (Thyroid Stimulating Hormone). You may have a doctor that will test T4, the inactive but necessary thyroid hormone. These two markers only show a part of the puzzle, leaving important pieces missing. TSH is the "Messenger" sent from the pituitary gland that is located in the center of the brain. Testing TSH is needed to tell us how well the messaging system is working to the thyroid. It can also inform the practitioner how well the thyroid gland is receiving and processing the message sent from the pituitary. However, you still have not tested the actual thyroid function.

Once TSH delivers the message to the thyroid, the thyroid gland will make T4. T4 should then work to convert into an active form of thyroid hormone called T3. There are different ways the body stores and uses T3. Some of T4 may convert to Reverse T3, which is the storage and survival form for emergencies, but ultimately, if this process is working well, it will convert to the active form T3 which will then be delivered into the cells where needed.

In my opinion, thyroid testing is one of the biggest failures in medicine because the standard testing is just TSH. As you can see, the process of the conversion of T4 to T3 is what's most important to regulate your metabolism, control body temperature, influence heart and digestive rate, and help with calcium regulation. If there is a glitch in this process, there are natural ways to support proper thyroid function.

Pro Tip: 80% of your thyroid conversion of T4 to T3 is done through the liver and 20% is done through the gut. We start all of our wellness to weight loss patients on a simple and effective detoxification program including our anti-inflammatory diet, supplements and addressing low-grade infections. You will want to detoxify the gut, liver, kidneys and the bowels and incorporate a diet that reduces inflammation.

Vitamin D is a hormone! Vitamin D is another significant hormone that is often underestimated for its ability to assist in overall well-being and immune health. Having sufficient levels of Vitamin D can be one of the quickest ways to start feeling better. It's one of the best antioxidants to help protect you from infections, support brain, skin, and hair health, helps to reduce symptoms of autoimmune, risks of Cancer, helps with sinus issues, thyroid function and menopausal symptoms, promotes healthy teeth, and lungs and helps repair muscles after being stressed. High levels of cortisol will cause you to lose Vitamin D fast and the pancreas needs Vitamin D in the making of insulin. It also helps to lower blood pressure and supports the liver which in turn can reduce your risk of insulin resistance, fatty liver and inflammation of the liver.

Pro Tip: With the many blood labs we have reviewed over the years, we've only seen a few that fall within the healthy range of 80-100 ng/mL. Don't assume you're getting enough Vitamin D because the sun is out. Some of the most deficient people live in the sunny states of Florida and California. Also, even if your Vitamin D is high it doesn't mean your body is absorbing it so there are many other tests to run. Another very important tip is due to chronobiology, we believe it is very beneficial to take your Vitamin D after 4:00 p.m. It is a fat soluble so taking it with your meal can also help absorption.

The old adage of eat less, exercise more has been proven to be wrong and most likely detrimental. We now know eating less (long-term restricted calories) can ultimately slow down the metabolism making it harder to lose weight. As stated above, what we eat and when we eat is most important. Exercising more i.e. (extreme workouts, boot camps, cross-fit, etc.) may not be the most beneficial forms of exercise for everyone, especially if overweight with underlying health issues. Pushing your body beyond the available resources is stressful on the body. If you are a stress bucket and you work out like a crazy person, your body is going to need a lot more resources to protect your muscles, bones and the many organs, glands and systems running the show. This can be a vicious cycle of yo-yo dieting causing weight loss plateaus, insulin resistance and even muscle wasting.

When you are not seeing significant results on the scale or the way your clothes fit to justify such intense and demanding workouts, and restriction of calories, one has to pause. Like all other systems, we believe testing is just as important for diet and exercise. Though the world has only scratched the surface in genetics, there is a lot of information now available so we can learn how our bodies are uniquely designed to operate, which is why genetic testing is a valuable part of our program.

Changing your mindset is essential when it comes to losing weight. It is important to cultivate a positive and determined mindset that focuses on long-term success rather than the quick fixes. Believing in your ability to overcome social pressure, obstacles, and get through life events can help you stay motivated and committed throughout your weight loss journey. Additionally, adapting a mindset that prioritizes self-care and self-compassion can help you navigate setbacks and avoid the negative self-talk. Focus on the process, not just on the outcome. Celebrate small victories with positive healthy rewards: like a new outfit, a massage, coffee with a friend. Choose to reward your good behavior with a good behavior, not a bad one. Use the scale as an accountability partner but remember, it may not always show a loss. Don't let this ruin your positive mindset and stop the actions you've already taken towards being healthier and losing those excess pounds. Focus more on the non-scale victories such as your increased energy levels, better sleep, mood improvement, and how well your clothes are fitting!

Cultivate a support system by surrounding yourself with encouraging family and friends who share similar aspirations and have a positive influence on helping you reach your goals. Set realistic goals, and stay consistent with healthy habits, to create lasting changes in your lifestyle to achieve optimal health and sustainable weight loss.

Remember, weight loss is a journey that involves both your physical and mental well-being. By adopting a positive mindset and embracing healthy habits, you can create lasting changes that will support your efforts! Practice mindful eating: Pay attention to your body's hunger and fullness cues and eat with intention and awareness. Slow down while eating, put the fork down between each bite, take a breath and savor the flavor.

Pro Tip: Getting your mindset right and reducing emotional stress can play a major role in our ability to maintain a healthy weight. When you find yourself in a stressful moment do yourself a favor, and LAUGH! Just Laugh! I know it sounds silly, but this silly action triggers an increase in endorphins creating more oxygen to the brain, improving a salty-sour or sad mood and you will even burn calories!

To summarize Wellness to Weight loss remember you get healthy to lose weight, not lose weight to get healthy. Don't wait for that dreaded diagnosis of a terminal illness. Wouldn't you have regrets for not taking your health more seriously? It seems as though more women than men focus on weight loss over their health, but the reality is, if your initial focus is on wellness your body can maintain a healthy weight. Excess weight is often just a symptom or side effect of something not right in the body. Women also seem to spend a fortune on their appearance but feel guilty when it comes to spending money on their health. When the reality is, it's the most important thing they can do for their appearance and slow down the aging process. The longer you wait the harder and more detrimental it could be, and at what cost? There's no better time than now to make your health and weight loss goals a top priority. I know now I'm grateful for that devastating glance in the mirror that pushed me to take my first step. Now I am blessed with the opportunity to work remotely with people all over the country helping them to also feel fantastic, look their best, and love the bodies they're in.

In the end, I want you to be able to look in the mirror, smile and know exactly HOW YOU GOT HERE!

If you would like to learn more about our Wellness To Weight Loss Programs, detoxes, DNA testing, take a Free Health Assessment to determine recommended baseline customized vitamins, tips or schedule your Free 15-minute discovery call visit: www.WellnessToWeightLoss.info

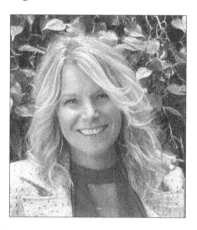

Dr. Angela Rahm, Board Certified Naturopathic Doctor. She specializes in full body health, safe and easy detoxing and long-lasting weight loss protocols. She works with people all over the country to help them get off the vicious cycle of yo-yo dieting, hormonal chaos, lack of energy and motivation so they can get their lives back and love the body they are in!

CHAPTER 9:

Trial and Error Health

By: Sydney Torres, FDNP

I was not going to share what I'm about to reveal to you in this chapter.

I felt like it was a "me only" problem and nobody else would really care about what some random girl was going through and experiencing. I kept silent, put on that front of "I can handle anything", but deep down inside I was falling apart. I thought to myself "I don't have time for a breakdown. I'm busy taking care of children, a spouse, and making sure my household is running smoothly."

Before I get deeper into my story, how about a proper introduction. Who I am, what I do, and why I do it. Hi, hello nice to meet you, I'm Sydney Torres a certified functional nutrition health practitioner and certified functional blood chemistry analyst. I do this because I no longer want to see anyone suffer and not get their health problems resolved. I no longer want to stand by and have others hear there's nothing wrong with them when deep down inside they know something is not right. I am here to be of service to you, to help, to educate, uplift, inspire, and most importantly bring your health back into balance so you can start living life on your own terms.

So this is where it began, on the top of my head. I was blessed with beautiful thick hair ever since I was born. I was always complimented on my hair's luster; I knew it looked good until I noticed more hair in my brush. The shower drain would fill up quickly getting clogged with strands upon strands of my hair. I remember it so clearly, one day as I was parting my hair, I noticed the edge of my hairline was completely gone.

I initiated code red getting my primary doctor to squeeze me into an appointment as soon as possible. The first thing that was done was a blood test. Once I got the results, I was told everything was "normal" except for a low white blood cell count and to watch my glucose numbers. I was told to come back in six weeks to get another blood draw. My doctor had zero idea why my hair was falling out. I felt like I was given no guidance, no answers, and no solutions. From there I made an appointment with a dermatologist which proved to be another dead end. The answers and solutions were presented in the form of prescriptions. Not wanting to medicate my issues away, I knew there was a better way to heal my body. I felt like a dog chasing its own tail going around in circles, feeling the frustrations of just wanting to feel well, physically, and mentally. As time went on other crazy symptoms started popping up. My hair went from falling out to bald spots throughout. I had inflammation in my hip and legs that made it hard to sleep or even get comfortable. I had unexplained skin rashes that took not one, not two, but three doctors called into the examination room looking and staring at every inch of my naked body while I just sat there hoping for an answer, just to hear, "I don't know, we have never seen this before."

Things slowly got worse over time. From having heart palpitations to having a cardiologist run every test imaginable. The anxiety and panic attacks that seemed to come out of nowhere, along with chronic fatigue, small intestinal bacterial overgrowth aka SIBO, H. Pylori which is a nasty bacteria that burrows inside the lining of the stomach, heavy metal toxicity, and estrogen dominance. All of my symptoms read like a long shopping list, but I still had to do my best to function as a mother, wife, friend, and an employee which proved to be a challenge within itself.

I got exhausted from doctors telling me, "your test is normal," and sending me on my way. That's when I decided to take things into my own hands. I figured, I'm smart, I've got a bachelor's degree—I can figure this out. So that's what I did. I decided at that moment to take my health and power back. I spent the next two and a half years learning about functionalmedicine, nutrition, and functional blood chemistry analysis. Getting every certification under the sun, I was determined to crack my own health case.

My health challenge started with my hair falling out then progressed into a long shopping list of symptoms. The mistake I made was making all of my symptoms the main focus. Instead of trying to eliminate each and every symptom, I should've been asking myself, "what is going on inside my body that is causing different signs and symptoms to manifest up to the surface?" The mistakes I made can be common for people to make when trying to solve their health issues.

During my health trial-and-error phase I hit the University of YouTube and Dr. Google really hard. I researched each and every condition I had like a mad scientist. I went to almost every local herb store within a twenty-five mile radius. I used the herbs to make hair tonics, DIY shampoos and conditioners. I even purchased a juicer and made green juice every single morning and tried the latest and greatest diet trends at the time. I was doing so many different things hoping and praying that my next pursuit would be the key to make me feel good again. I thought to myself "Why is all of this effort not working?" Being caught in the cycle of health trial-and-error happens to so many of us and to be honest, I thought this approach to health was the only way. I accepted it and thought I was going to be this way forever, until I really saw it up close and personal.

I worked for six years as a certified nursing assistant in a hospital. Working in all the departments from the emergency room, med-surg, psych unit, and the ICU. I started to notice a common theme. Can you guess? Yes, the vicious cycle of health trial-and-error. Not only was I caught up in my own cycle but seeing my patients caught up really helped me realize this issue wasn't only me and went extremely deep. This made me even more determined to figure out why. Why are people trying everything from A-Z and not seeing any real shifts within their health?

What I observed was this: patients would get admitted, stay a few days, and then get discharged. Within a few weeks the same group of patients would be admitted again for the same health complaint. Staff would refer to these patients as "frequent fliers." I asked practically the entire hospital staff including the attending physicians, "Why do these same patients keep coming back and for the exact same thing?" No one could provide any real answers to me, besides "these things just happen" or "things just happen with age." Refusing to accept that as a concrete answer my quest continued to seek the real reason for what was going on not only for myself but everyone else who is struggling with any sort of health challenge.

I was first introduced to functional medicine while I was attending the Institute for Integrative Nutrition. The ideas and the model structure just made sense to me and that's when I started to have the paradigm shift from standard health care to functional care. I just felt like this was the answer to all my ailing health conditions if I could only learn more. After graduating from IIN I enrolled in Functional Nutrition Alliance School and learned even more. I was so determined to feel good in my body again and drop all these chronic conditions like a bad habit. While attending Functional Nutrition Alliance I was introduced to functional testing like hormone testing, hair testing, and reading blood labs. After experiencing on more than one occasion not having my test results and blood labs interpreted correctly, I had the mindset of, I could do it better. This led me to enroll at Functional Diagnostic Nutrition where I was taught how to properly use functional lab testing and interpret results. The more I learned and educated myself, the more I realized why so many people were not getting results when it came to their issues.

What keeps not only myself, my patients, and the rest of the world coming back to the same starting point, which is not getting health issues resolved? The more I learned about functional health care, the more answers started to get revealed. One of the principle foundations is uncovering the hidden underlying root causes of what is going on within the body. Let me put it like this, if you were to plant a tree you would provide top quality soil so the tree's roots would be supported. The top quality soil would have vital nutrients, plenty of water and sunshine. The roots in return would be able to grow and produce strong tree branches that were full of beautiful vibrant green leaves. To answer the question of what was going on with myself and kept my patients returning to the hospital multiple times- our health issues were being addressed at the incorrect level.

Let me go back to the tree analogy. If the tree you planted was sick with brown leaves that were dry and brittle would you simply cut off the branches expecting the tree to thrive again? Cutting off the branches would be a temporary solution and a quick fix. In order for the tree to regain vitality again, the soil must be addressed. Not addressing the underlying root causes, will keep you stuck in the ugly health cycle of trial and error.

Ask yourself the question: Am I ready to get off this revolving merry-go-round? Hopefully you've answered yes. Let me tell you some ways to stop the cycle of health trial-and-error and get out for good.

Here are some very important questions so you can determine if you've been caught in the cycle of health trial-and-error:

1) Your cabinet looks like your local health food store or local GNC
2) You're not getting better despite trying multiple things
3) You've been to multiple providers with no answers, guidance, or solutions
4) Your medication list is growing
5) You feel like each body part is being addressed separately and not the whole you
6) Your provider is treating your symptoms and not getting to the underlying root causes.

If you've answered yes to any of the reasons above, chances are you're stuck. Feeling trapped and not making progress with reaching health goals can be beyond frustrating. I would know because I've been there myself.

So, what is the difference between standard health care vs the functional health care model? Standard health care examines individual symptoms and assumes that they're related to various body parts. Standard health care prescribes medication or medical procedures to alleviate symptoms and to eliminate illness. Functional health care focuses on restoring health instead of merely eliminating illness. Giving the body what it needs in order to regain balance and function correctly.

What is missing from standard health care that makes not only myself and these patients frequently get caught in the vicious cycle of health trial-and-error? The standard medical approach focuses on treating and managing symptoms which can include surgery and pharmaceuticals. One of the ways to stop the cycle is to stop chasing symptoms. Does this sound like you? You visited several doctors and even specialists who simply prescribed medication to help with symptoms A,B, or C. You are on the fence about whether or not to take the pills. You start to get really frustrated and are desperate for relief, so you decide to go pick up that prescription from the pharmacy. You do get relief, but it only lasts for a short while.

Please understand that symptoms are not the problem but the result of the problem. The symptoms are a sign of a deeper underlying issue within the body. Over time new symptoms appear, and you start feeling worse and worse. Standard health care has made symptoms the target, and this is part of the reason why people aren't resolving their health complaints.

If only treating symptoms, there likely will not be a real shift in health. Becoming your own health advocate and educating yourself on other options starts to put more of the power back into your hands. Being supported by a practitioner who is prevention-oriented will make the journey easier. If you're not already familiar with the functional health model, I would like to introduce a different way to approach health and wellness. After working six years in a hospital which was focused around the sick care model, it was a breath of fresh air adopting the functional health care approach. Breaking free from the standard health care way of thinking really allowed me to take my laundry list of unresolved health complaints and start crossing them off. Once I really learned and started implementing this approach I thought, why isn't all of health care like this?

I would like to take a minute to paint the picture of the functional health care model, and the great benefits it can do for your personal well-being. The functional approach addresses the underlying root causes of dysfunction within the body. Functional practitioners look at each patient or client as a whole person and do not focus solely on one body part or body system. We understand that the body works as an entire system and never independently of itself. The functional approach considers factors like diet, genetics, lifestyle, environment, stress, personal relationships, exercise habits, emotional well-being and more. We look at the entire picture. We also understand that each person is bio-individual, and each health plan is tailored specifically for that individual.

I want to give you the keys to unlock your body's innate intelligence. I challenge you to think differently, be bold in your choices and not afraid to be open to new ideas and concepts. When it comes to suffering from unresolved health complaints, think about approaching it in a new way. Continuously doing something the same way is always going to yield the same results. As a society we have been so conditioned to think health is linear. We've been taught to take this pill to solve our body's problems. There is a better way, let me show you, if you are ready to get back to the life you deserve. Think of how good you will feel taking a vacation with family or friends. Having the energy to do your favorite activities. Energy for kids or grandkids. Finally, being able to enjoy those foods at your favorite restaurants. Now is the time to start thriving and not just surviving. Are you ready to stop doing what is not working? Change can be scary, but you must believe you can break through.

A common question I'm asked is, my blood labs came back "normal" and I still feel horrible. I know something is not right, I've tried everything and I'm about to give up. *What can I do?*

The existing blood labs you already have are full of answers and solutions. Before you go telling me your doctor has already looked at your blood labs and everything came back normal, "what makes you qualified to tell me anything different." This is a very good question, and I would like to unpack this right now.

I was very blessed to be trained and mentored by two of the best functional doctors who specialize in functional blood analysis. Dr. Kylie Burton and Dr. Dicken Weatherby.

It's important to lay some basic foundation, this way you'll have a better understanding. First, it's important to understand that blood lab results are based on reference ranges. Think of reference ranges as a set of values that have upper and lower limits. These ranges are used by health practitioners so they can interpret a patient's test results. The ranges also help show what a typical "normal" result looks like.

There are two types of Ranges. Standard Reference Ranges, which are used by standard health care, and Functional Reference Ranges which are used by practitioners who approach health from the holistic point of view.

Standard ranges are way too wide. Think of the distance between California and New York. Within that long distance a lot can go wrong. Keep in mind, the wider the range the more difficult it is to detect any health problems BEFORE it turns into disease. Now let's talk about Functional Ranges. These ranges are much tighter and based on "optimal" lab values. The values allow us to explore any imbalances before they can progress into something big and ugly. When you fall outside the range this means that something within the body is not functioning the way it should. Blood labs really do give insight on how the body is functioning.

When dysfunction starts this is the time where different symptoms will come up to the surface. It's at this point, you start to feel unwell. The cool thing about blood labs is we can see trends and patterns. We can see if a client is moving towards the direction of health or moving towards the direction of something unwanted.

To really show you the power of blood labs I will be sharing a few examples. I want to also point out that doctors read labs from the viewpoint of looking for disease. Functional practitioners read labs from the point of view of prevention and detect where the dysfunction lies and then make course corrections as needed through diet, lifestyle, mindset, and environment.

Before I came into the functional space I never considered what an asset blood labs could be. Labs were something that were routinely run for an annual check-up or for a sick visit with a health provider. Blood labs can provide valuable answers and solutions if the person knows how to interpret from a functional perspective. Learning blood labs from a functional point of view was a huge contributor to finding my hidden internal stressors. Not only was I able to finally crack my own health case but now I am able to be a health detective for others who are experiencing unresolved chronic health conditions.

Throughout my journey I often would hear the famous words, "everything is normal." I would like to share a few things I found in my so-called "normal" blood labs and I will make some clinical correlations. I will be referencing the lab that was taken when my health challenge started to appear.

Let me start with gastrointestinal function, aka gut health. When speaking about gut health think of a long tube running from the mouth to the anus. The G.I. is responsible for digestion and absorption of the food we eat. If the G.I. is not working properly, it can cause a host of cascading effects throughout the entire body system. In my case I was told everything looked good and was within the standard range. Going back and reviewing my old labs with my new detective skills, this is what I discovered, again I am reviewing this from a functional perspective.

All of the following markers were low: BUN marker, total protein, albumin, globulin and low alkaline phosphatase. So what does this mean? Instead of me trying to explain each and every marker it will be easier to provide the big picture of what was going on.

Here comes the big picture. Many assume that if they chew and swallow their food they will absorb it, this is not always true. One of the first places gut health takes place is within the stomach. The stomach's main job is to produce acidic digestive juices that are known as hydrochloric acid (HCL).

When we get stressed out and are in the fight or flight mode this shuts down HCL and enzyme production. If we don't get enough sleep, have a poor diet or don't get enough protein in the diet the same thing will happen. Being deficient in nutrients such as iron, zinc, and b-vitamins which are needed to make stomach acid. Without adequate stomach acid this can increase the risk for other issues like bacterial overgrowth, acid reflux, bloating, gas, gut infections, constipation, leaky gut, gallbladder issues, and much more. Going back to the above markers mentioned, I had low stomach acid.

Let me connect some dots here. Backing it up a little bit, let me give a little insight on what my diet and lifestyle was like back then. I was a hardcore vegan working the night shift at a hospital which was from 7pm-7am so my sleep was way off. Most of the time my stress level was a ten out of ten. Let's just say I was running in the red most of the time. Due to the low stomach acid, this was contributing to my food not properly being broken down. Stomach acid is needed for digestion and absorption of protein and vitamin B12 and other minerals. When the body can't break down and absorb its nutrients you can end up with undigested food and nutritional deficiencies. When the undigested food is left, it can ferment in the G.I tract which then can lead to bacterial overgrowth in the small intestines aka SIBO.

In my situation it got to the point where I was very deficient in minerals, vitamins, not getting enough protein through my vegan diet, lack of sleep, on top of the low stomach acid created the snowball effect. The snowball effect is a process that starts off small and then builds upon itself into something larger and more serious. My snowball turned into SIBO, H.Pylori, leaky gut and more. The whole point in sharing this with you is that my "snowball" could have been prevented had my initial labs been read from a functional viewpoint. Just think how many clues are lying in your labs that you were told were normal. Using regular targeted blood tests can help detect early stages of dysfunction. The body will be dysfunctional first before it gets to the diseased state. Some early stages of dysfunction can range from G.I. dysfunction, oxidative stress, toxicity, hormone and thyroid imbalances, neuroendocrine and blood sugar dysregulation just to name a few.

I would like to leave you with one last thought. Remember it's not just one thing that is contributing to your body's imbalance, it's usually many causative factors. When getting blood labs, think of each biomarker like a puzzle piece to your health. You have to have the correct pieces aka correct biomarkers ordered and the correct person interpreting your labs from a functional point of view this way the entire picture of what's going on can be seen.

Tired of not getting answers and solutions to your unresolved chronic health complaints and want a second opinion on your blood labs? Find me at the link below and sign up for a consultation and I can get you answers. You can find me at https://www.balancehealthnowvhc.com/beyond-normal-blood-labs

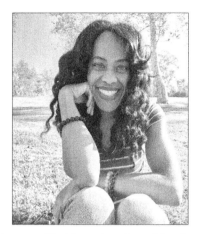

Sydney Torres is a certified functional nutrition health practitioner. After working six years as a certified nursing assistant in a hospital, she realized there was a better way to approach health and wellness. She now helps women with unresolved health complaints find answers and solutions within their so-called normal blood labs. She helps them so they can get back to enjoying life again. When she is not helping clients she enjoys taking road trips with her kids and family. She enjoys being silly, laughing and gardening and growing her own food.

CHAPTER 10:

Let's Make it Personal

By: Patty Jo Burress

A loyal client of mine walks into the shop one morning and looks just sad and beside herself. She says to me something has to change. I said, "what's going on?" She explains she had to go to the ER this weekend because she felt like she was having a heart attack. She said, "I had no energy, I couldn't breathe, I had sharp pains in my heart, I don't know." The doctor said I was very nutritionally deficient. I am so filled up with fluid I feel like I am going to burst. DJ was a frequently distressed caller begging for treatments at all hours for her chronic pain throughout her body. She had come in often for massages, infrared light therapy, & biofeedback. It all helped but just for a short time. She is about five-foot and 287 lbs. We had visited numerous times and she mentioned that if she could just lose some weight it would really help her. I encouraged her that when she was ready to make a few lifestyle changes I was ready to support her. She had to make the call. I had been trying to encourage DJ that we should team up and tackle some lifestyle issues for awhile. Her list of surgeries is a mile long. She had struggled with her weight, health, and emotional distress from past trauma. We are finding that many health conditions are caused by excess stress, negative emotions, and life traumas.

When we visited about it I could hear her fear of failure and frustration in her voice and body language. She had mentioned she had tried every diet and weight loss supplement on the market. Her sister and her even had bought some type of fat sucking device. I couldn't tell you

the name of it. All I know when she showed it to me it looked like they hadn't used it much and I told her that was a blessing she hadn't. You see like most fad diets and quick fix supplements

on the market it would help her lose some and it would all come back and then some. At this time I was launching my new personalized signature wellness pilot program and offered it to her. It was definitely a fit. She was very frightened that she was going to die and was going to do exactly what her doctor said. Which wasn't wrong. He told her she needed to change her

lifestyle or she wouldn't be here much longer, prescribed her some pills & gave her a couple

books to read and out the door she went.

DJ's Personalized Signature Wellness Plan

When setting up plans for my clients I believe one size does NOT fit all. I help assist you to find the mindset that will help achieve your personal goals. The body is made to heal itself if given the right tools. In this program I offer specialized testing, lifestyle change, biofeedback Therapies and other modalities. These help destress the body quickly which causes less dis-ease in the body. We offer exceptional client guidance, support, and accountability by blending two different biofeedback devices with health coaching, PFC Plate, InLight Therapy, LymphStar Pro, IonCleanse, Massage, Cranial Sacral, and nutritional supplements homeopathy, Lifewave Patches & herbal remedies.

If you are a client that walks through the doors of Knead It or Knot, all of the following modalities are in your tool kit. If you are a remote client we will help find someone in your area to help you receive the needed therapies that we cannot do on-line. We do our best to personalize your container to make your health journey a success.

BodyMind Coaching

The heart felt coaching is all about helping people to eat, sleep, move, & release stress optimally so they can live up to their fullest potential! It is an excellent option for anyone motivated and ready to release weight, improve their energy and mood, get to the bottom of what is going on in their body, and take responsibility for their health.

DJ and I sat down together and found clarity on what her goals were and what she thought she needed to change. She mentioned how she was disabling herself, how she was eating and how she felt. We talked about what it was going to take to make the change and what her first steps were going to be. She already knew all the answers to what needed to be done to feel better and be healthy. She just needed the support to organize them.

Quantum Biofeedback

Biofeedback is a state-of-the-art technology designed to help strip away the layers of stress and balance the body, mind and spirit. We deal with only what the body is ready to deal with. This technology produces a detailed scan that helps us identify what is stressing the body. The power of this process is gaining a new understanding of the client a little at a time. This modality can be done in person or remote.

What are the benefits of Biofeedback?
- Quicker, more effective relaxation
- Greater sense of well-being
- Improved sleep quality

- Reduced stress and nervousness
- Reduced anger, fear, apprehension and gloominess
- Decreased generalized, specific, or headache pain
- Better muscle/joint mobility and coordination/Reduction of Inflammation
- Improved general flexibility
- Enhanced athletic performance
- Heightened mental clarity, memory and attention
- Improved overall health
- Pain Reduction
- Anti-Aging

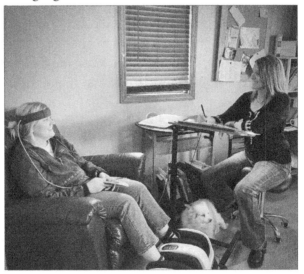

The PFC Plate

The PFC plate showed amazing results for DJ in just one month. She lost forty-four pounds and her inflammation decreased. The PFC plate plate helped DJ make behavioral change simply by helping her create new nutritional habits. First thing first, DJ went home and cleared her house of all processed foods. The nice thing about this plate is it helps you choose the appropriate serving sizes and shows what foods should be eaten along with portion size. It is conveniently listed on the plate for your three main meals with a balanced snack in between. We did personalize this for her. The biofeedback devices found what her stressors were in her eating habits. Dairy, gluten, pork and surprise, sugar were her top stressors. You see when eating the right balance and amounts of proteins, fats and carbohydrates, you balance blood sugar, restore homeostasis, and ignite your metabolism.

Whether your goal is weight loss, gaining lean muscle, or simply renewing your health, the PFC plate will teach you to nourish your body supporting your goals and leaving you feeling energized. We personalize this to your needs and incorporate fasting and the lifestyle that best fits your body's needs.

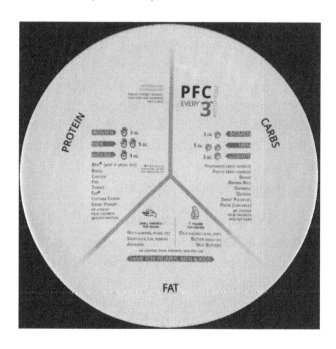

Let's Take a Look at Your Bloodwork

DJ brought her full CBC with differential to our meeting. We sat down to analyze it and found out her blood sugar was an issue and was the culprit to many other issues she was having. Her blood sugar, A1C and Cholesterol Panel were all high. Her A1C was at 10.7. Her glucose was over 600. Let me repeat what the doctor said to her. You must change your lifestyle or you're not going to be here any longer! You have too much sugar and too much fat, he repeated.

So the first thing we did was start on Systemic Formulas Synulin along with the prep phase to help support the body. The healthy fats along with the kidney & liver support is just what her body needed. MORS helped her energy level. We also added DV3 to help with inflammation.

Let's remember she was eating too much sugar and too many unhealthy fats. She felt so sick...all she wanted to do was sleep and had no energy. She felt like she was disabling herself and they had run lots of tests.

We used her updated blood work and biofeedback sessions throughout her journey to help customize and support her nutritional/ supplement needs. In this client-case we used the Pre-phase, Body Phase, Brain phase and Cellular Vitality in her package. She liked the kits.

They are all packaged and conveniently.

What is InLight Therapy?

InLight Medical LED light therapy systems are different from any other pain relief remedy you've tried. LED light therapy supports the body's natural healing processes to reduce pain and inflammation. Wavelengths of multicolored light, known as polychromatic light, deliver unique benefits that our bodies can only receive from low-level light therapy. InLight is able to penetrate within 100 millimeters into the body. DJ used this often for pain relief from a chronic pain and a few injuries she had. We want to take the best care of your body every day, InLight therapy can easily support effortless wellness. InLight Medical LED light therapy devices are FDA cleared for increasing circulation and reducing pain.

What are the benefits of InLight Therapy?

InLight's gentle, pulsing LED light wavelengths increase circulation to relieve pain and rejuvenate the entire body by activating ATP within the cells. Although gentle, silent and cool to the touch, low-level light therapy is naturally effective on a cellular level. And unlike painkillers, not only does light therapy relieve pain, it also addresses the underlying condition by stimulating the body's innate healing abilities.

Many people with symptoms associated with the following conditions experience positive results from using LED light therapy:

- Neck pain
- Back Pain
- Leg pain
- Shoulder pain
- Knee pain
- Ankle problems
- Arthritis
- Inflammation and swelling
- Bone spurs
- Bone fractures
- Bruises
- Burns
- Carpal tunnel
- Tennis elbow
- Healing wounds

- Peripheral neuropathy
- Tight muscles
- PTSD
- Anti-Aging
- Hair rejuvenation

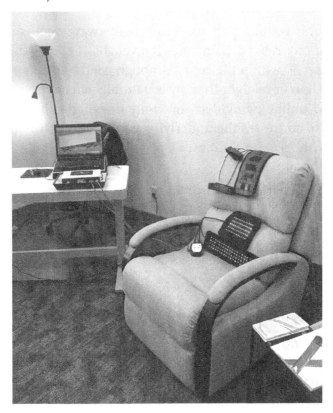

LymphStar®Pro Fusion

Knead It or Knot uses the LymphStar and Ionic Foot bath to help open the detoxification outlets, accelerates detoxification of your tissues and increases lymphatic circulation. We are dedicated to helping you feel better by addressing what is so often overlooked: your lymphatic system. During the end of phase one of your personalized action plan we add these two modalities to prepare and support your body for your next step. The detoxification phase can make us feel sluggish and just sometimes yucky. When using these modalities it makes the detoxification phase easier by providing you relaxation, emotional balance and feelings of well-being with increased energy.

The lymphatic system transports and cleanses every cell and organ in the body. It is the pathway for toxins to be removed from the body and plays a key role in immune function as the white blood cells are transported through the lymph. Using Lymphstar and footbath aids in remove this congestion, allowing more nutrients to be supplied to the cells, removing toxins, and increasing immune function.

The Lymphstar uses subtle vibrational energy to encourage the clearing and release of accumulated fluid, toxins, and proteins which reside in the interstitial tissue spaces. As such it emits "information" to the energy field of the cells via harmonics of sound and frequencies of light. It produces this information by way of something called "noble gas ionization." There is a long tradition of research into the energetic effects of these noble gasses. An optimal mixture of xenon and argon is enclosed in a Pyrex glass tube. The gasses are excited by electrical currents. An energy field, or plasma, then radiates from the tube onto the skin and is conducted through the entire bio-energy system. The Lymphstar is applied by placing the transmission head, or heads on the skin. Use of the instrument on the body is followed by manual lymphatic drainage. Lymphstar is effective for breast health, pain syndromes, edema, immune issues, postoperative and injury healing, and rapid aging, low collagen formation of the skin, hormone balancing and to decrease stress. The therapy improves edemas, fibrotic conditions, and swollen lymph nodes. Some conditions reported to have benefited from therapy include breast lumps, inflammation, chronic pain, joint aches, muscle pain, sports injuries, post surgery allergies, sinus, respiratory problems, headaches, prostate problems, hormone imbalance and chronic female conditions, dental trauma and chronic problems, heavy metal toxicity, neuromuscular trauma, immune and fatigue syndromes and promotes drainage of excess fluid.

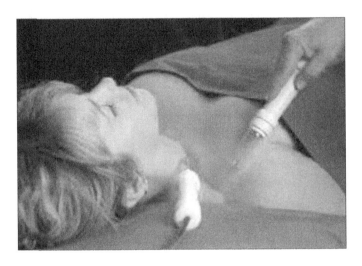

IönCleanse Foot Bath

The IonCleanse® by AMD helps the body detox through the healing power of ions. Negatively and positively ions, because of their powerful charge, cleanse the body more effectively than any other method of detox. It is a unique total body detox using electrical frequencies that have the ability to be in contact with a living system without any harsh side effects.

How Does it Work?

Three simple steps

- First, the clean current interaction with the warm water helps to bring out a relaxation response in the body.

- Second, this current works by ionizing the water molecule, splitting the H2O into Oh- & ht ions. These ions act like billions of tiny magnets in the water do create the initial draw of oppositely charged toxins from the body.
- Third & Lastly, the relaxation effect experienced during the foot bath produces an ongoing detoxification release for the body for three to five days. Clients may go to the bathroom more, sweat more & we always suggest that you stay hydrated during this process.

We have seen great results by supporting our metabolic, neurological, endocrine, immune, and digestive systems during the detox process. If you experiencing fatigue, cognitive dysfunction, brain fog, thyroid, adrenal, hormones, ADH, viral, fungal, and bacterial infections, dysbiosis, leaky gut, malabsorption, heavy metals, glyphosate, & food intolerances, the IonCleanse will be incorporated into your program.

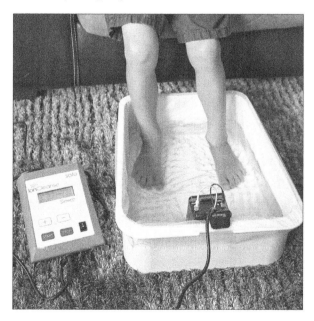

Cranial Sacral

We use Craniosacral Therapy for people suffering from headaches, chronic pain, TMJ, chronic

fatigue, depression, anxiety, dizziness, vertigo and sleep challenges to name just some medical conditions. Sometimes people are struggling with past traumas to the head or have had a traumatic event in their life that they have not dealt with and have opened up and released that energy that has kept them stuck in their path to healing.

Craniosacral Therapy also helps with:
- Migraine and tension headaches
- Temporomandibular joint pain (TMJ)
- Neck, shoulder girdle, and lower back pain
- Post-traumatic injuries of the head and neck and whiplash
- Fibromyalgia
- Chronic fatigue syndrome
- Problems with alertness, concentration, or memory
- Anxiety and stress-related problems

Craniosacral therapy is a gentle hands-on technique that uses a light touch to examine membranes and movements of the fluids in and around the central nervous system. Relieving tension in the central nervous system promotes a feeling of well-being by eliminating pain and boosting health and immunity.

The technique can also be used anywhere on the body to release restrictions in the connective tissue to bring back rhythm there and to relieve any pain. Craniosacral Therapy seeks to locate and remove restrictions throughout the body's systems. Corrections to these systems are addressed through light touch, time, energy and intention.

Massage Therapy

We offer over twenty-three years of combined experience in bodywork. In addition to receiving your full session time we customize your session to fit you. Therapeutic massage therapy is a wonderful addition with all of the modalities in your action plan. It increases blood flow, increases relaxation, and promotes an overall sense of well being.

It can help to relieve pain in muscles, open areas around the lymph nodes, and help a person to feel more like themselves again.

Indications for Massage:
- Back Pain
- Headaches
- Whiplash
- Pelvic Pain
- Neck Pain
- Stress
- Chronic Pain
- Disc Problems
- Migraines
- Fibromyalgia
- Chronic Fatigue Syndrome
- Adhesions
- Carpal Tunnel
- Jaw Pain (TMJ)

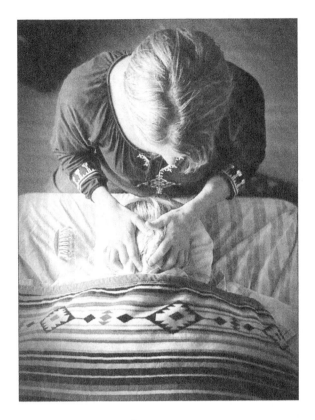

DJ's Journey

"I am so thankful to get my life back. In August I never dreamt that by December I would have lost 72 lbs. I was so excited that I could wear a large coat again. My shirts now look like dresses. Yes, I did it the healthy way. When April hit I was down a total of 96 lbs. I have maintained it and I know I still have a long way to go yet. But I know what steps I have to take. I feel like I am living a whole different life. People don't realize how you bog yourself down. It was like someone opened up the door and I felt free. My energy level has changed tremendously. I can easily go up and down three flights of stairs without being out of breath. My husband is so very thankful. He often says I am so glad my wife is back. It has made our marriage stronger. He no longer has to drag me out of bed.

The little things are easy now. I would be in the vehicle and drop something and couldn't pick it up. I said *ooh, ooh* when I dropped something on the floor I couldn't pick it up. I would just look over at my husband and say ooh ooh. My husband and I would just laugh at myself. I am always afraid to bend down and kneel with the thought that I am not going to be able to get back up. I can do that now without pain. I go to get a massage for maintenance instead of being in pain. My knee, back, and sciatic pain have disappeared. When we first started I was encouraged that movement is a needed tool. When we started my body would not allow me to do that. As the months went on we added small movements I could achieve without failure. I feel confident enough now that I am ready for the next level. I am not at my goal weight yet but

I can move! I am ready to firm up by doing some lifting and adding more movement. My blood sugar and A1C are approved by my doctor. Remember I was a 10.7. It is currently at a 6.8. My doctor is proud that it is at a healthy level now. My mindset, lifestyle change, and maybe learning that eating my vegetables out of a can was not reaching my nutritional needs. The supplements I am taking and the PFC plate designed for my action plan have helped me reach my nutritional needs."

With these holistic approaches, our clients experience improved health and quality of life.

DJ has shared her journey with her sister who has been on Metformin for ten years. Sharing her knowledge of how to eat and some of Systemic Formulas Products have changed her life.

Her doctor recently took her off of her Metformin.

Here are a couple pictures of DJ and her sister. These pictures are one year apart.

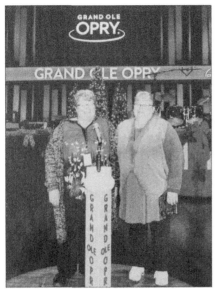 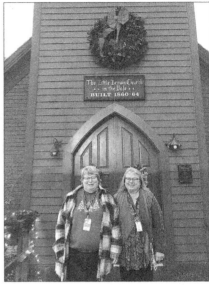

I'd love to see if I can help you too! You can find me on social media at https://www.facebook.com/KneadItOrKnotMassage-Therapy or www.pattyjoburress@gmail.com

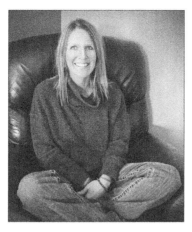

Hi, I am **Patty Jo.**

Some people call me PJ. I have two teenage boys and a kind, loving and supportive husband. I am an animal lover. We have horses, dogs, cats, goats, and of course cattle. We live on a cattle ranch northwest of Isabel, SD. We enjoy living out in the country and living the western lifestyle. We spend most of our extra time on the rodeo trail. We all enjoy the rodeo and going to ropings. It's a family affair.

I have been in the holistic health industry for twenty-three years. I love my business, as I never quit learning, and helping people fills my cup. I am passionate about helping my clients as we guide them toward improved wellness by owning their own health, no band-aid solutions, & looking at you as an entire person.

CHAPTER 11:

From Wheelchair to Walking

By: Kristie Hess-Newton

Have you ever wondered, *"how did I get here?"*

I did. A lot. And I've had plenty of reasons, over the years, to ask that question of my life.

The important part of my Health Journey started when I was about twenty-eight years old. At that time, I had been married for four years and together we had a four-year-old daughter, Hanna, and a one-year-old son, Jacob. The episodes started that Spring. I found myself becoming increasingly fatigued, my body literally collapsing, for no apparent reason. The only way I could describe my condition was… I had no strength. My legs felt like wet noodles, and my body felt as if it had been opened from the top and sand had been poured in until there was no more room. Each arm, each leg seemed to weigh a hundred pounds and my head was a 50-pound bowling ball that took every ounce of my strength to keep atop my shoulders. I simply couldn't carry the weight of my own body anymore.

"How did I get here?"

As I worked to piece together my health history, I knew I'd been diagnosed with Mononucleosis during my elementary school years, and again while in high school. Commonly referred to as "Mono," or the "Kissing Disease" (due to the ease of contracting it through the exchange of saliva), this was a viral condition typically caused by exposure and overgrowth of the Epstein-Barr virus (EBV) within a weakened immune system. It can lead to some troubling conditions, but with proper management and enough rest, the virus typically goes dormant within the recovery period, and a semblance of health returns. When I was twenty-six and working as a Cardiac Specialty Tech at our local hospital, my third episode was triggered by a human bite. The "worst bite I'd ever seen", claimed the ER doc who treated me. An elderly dementia patient I was assisting believed I was breaking into her home, and, in her addled state, bit a chunk from my arm! The physical, and likely emotional, trauma brought on my latest re-emergence of EBV.

Of course, at that time I had no idea the extent to which this virus would soon come to rule my life.

"How did I get here?"; "Why am I SO tired, so extremely fatigued, all the time?" ; "Why do I feel so heavy?" I asked doctor after doctor, then specialist after specialist. The consensus was that, although the test results showed that I had the EBV in my system, this shouldn't be the cause of my current issues.

"Your blood work looks normal." Because blood tests are the typical first step utilized today by most medical doctors to diagnose illness and guide the treatment decisions.

So, I was given the most popular diagnoses at the time for conditions that presented with vague symptoms and no easily defined disease processes: Chronic Fatigue Syndrome and Fibromyalgia. Basically, being told my exceptional exhaustion had a name, as did my near-constant muscle pain. I was sent on my way with a cocktail of medications, none of which worked to ease my suffering, or return me to a functional state. I woke up with Ritalin (an amphetamine, or "upper") and I relied on sleeping pills ("downers") to allow me to sleep. I took pain medication to get myself through the day. But nothing "fixed" me. I was twenty-eight-years-old, and I had less ability to care for myself than did a newborn baby. I was a mother of an infant and a toddler and I couldn't even handle my own needs. Not the least bit of an exaggeration, I was literally sleeping eighteen to twenty hours a day, every day and yet I was Still. Always.Tired. I can still remember the day I woke up, made my way to the living room couch, and promptly fell back to sleep until 2:30 in the afternoon. Mortified, I apologized to my sweet babies, "Mama's SO sorry! I didn't even get you two breakfast or lunch!" I slept right through both mealtimes.

"It's okay, Mommy. I got Jacob and me dry cereal for breakfast and made peanut butter sandwiches when we got hungry for lunch."

Hanna always knew how to step up and help mom when she was needed. And for that, I am eternally grateful. But no four-year-old should have to make meals for her little brother because Mom can't function enough to get up off the couch. That's not how life is supposed to work.

We were SO fortunate to have amazing family and friends who would come over to help when they could. Friends took on a rotation of house cleaning and cooking chores, so our family could survive. My mother came over to help me care for Hanna and Jacob. It even fell to her to help me shower, because I could collapse at a moment's notice, making showers dangerous. It was literally not safe for the children to be left alone in my care. I couldn't handle it.

Over the next few years, I submitted myself to numerous spinal taps, X-rays and ultrasounds, MRI's, CT scans, and every other test imaginable. The doctors found a few irregularities pointing to

Multiple Sclerosis, a potentially disabling disease of the brain and spinal cord that is caused by an attack of the immune system, targeting the protective sheath (myelin) that covers the nerves that run throughout the entire body. MS disrupts the communication between the brain and the rest of the body and could certainly account for my inability to function. But it was thought that, with me in my twenties, I was too young to have contracted MS, therefore my Neurologist was not comfortable assigning this diagnosis at the time, adopting a more "wait and see" approach. So, I continued to be treated for my symptoms of pain, weakness, and fatigue.

And time marched on. When I was thirty-one years old, I had my third child. A beautiful, and surprising blessing we named Samuel. For so many reasons, none the least of which was the complete resolution of my symptoms that began during my pregnancy. The doctors explained to us that, while pregnant, one of two things typically happens to a patient with my presentation. They either relapse with increasing symptoms, or they improve. Luckily for our family, my symptoms improved. I felt a return of energy and my health rebounded significantly. I was convinced I'd been healed of whatever illness had attacked me. That God had chosen to work a miracle in my life and restored me to complete health. Since I was now a stay-at-home mom, with three children, we decided to homeschool Hanna and Jacob. With my new-found vigor, more gratitude than most young moms get to experience, and a strong desire to "give back" due to my renewed health, we decided to become a foster family. After a few short-term opportunities, our precious two-year-old Jeremiah came into our lives... and stayed. Soon, we became a family of seven, when our last baby, a three-day-old baby girl named Sera, made our family complete. By the age of thirty-three, I had three biological children and two beautiful bonus babies, all under the age of eight.

So, my life got back on track, I was a home-schooling, stay-at-home mom of five fabulous kids. Life was Great. Church was fantastic. However, my marriage had started to bear the brunt of the years of illness, and the battle to regain my health. I was making things work as best I could, but I was mentally and emotionally struggling.

Suddenly, my feet got swept out from under me and in the blink of an eye, my illness returned. With a vengeance. I began collapsing while trying to walk, suffering extreme body weakness and pain throughout every muscle. The stress was unbearable. Money was tight, prescription costs were piling up, and we had no insurance, as my husband was self-employed, and I was no longer working outside the home. Soon, I could no longer function, and took to scooting myself around the house on my rolling office chair, unable to trust my body to bear my own weight on a regular basis. When Hanna was ten, she had to help me bathe in the sink in our half-bath downstairs, as I could no longer make it up to the full bathroom. I went months without an actual shower. The stairs were more than I could handle in my weakened state. I couldn't cook. I had to give up cleaning my home. My Mother tried her hardest to help, but she had been diagnosed with Dementia in the interim and was beginning to show signs of her own struggles. My friends continued to be amazing and kept us going with their love and assistance. They would take turns babysitting our kids so that I could sleep and tend to the basics.

Along with the worsening of my previous symptoms, soon the vision in my right eye faltered, and then was gone entirely. Adding an Ophthalmologist to my ever-growing list of doctors, we finally got the answers we needed.

After studying the myriad of tests he'd run, to try and determine why I'd suddenly gone blind in one eye, he asked the question that dropped my heart to the floor, yet gave me immense relief, all at the same time.

"Has anyone ever told you that you have Multiple Sclerosis?"

"YES! My Neurologist thought it was a possibility, but I was so young at the time…"

And so, it was confirmed. After almost ten years of fighting this monster, it finally had a name. Not "just" Fibromyalgia, or Chronic Fatigue Syndrome. Those words described merely two symptoms of a complex disease process. Multiple Sclerosis. The Granddaddy of them all. The complete loss of the myelin sheath of my right optic nerve was the determining factor in allowing for this official diagnosis. In my attempts to add MS treatment to my regimen, I had to find a new Neurologist, as my previous doctor was no longer practicing in our area.

MS meds added to our drug inventory, we experimented until we found what we hoped, my new Neurologist and I, was the right med for me. It took a few tries to find something that was workable. We struggled and cobbled our way through the next few years. Our family, our friends, the doctors, and God. We all did the best we could, but as my quality of life lessened with each passing day, the burden grew heavier as well.

I was no longer the Mom I wanted to be. I wasn't the Wife I needed to be, nor was I the Friend I longed to be. And according to MS, I never would be. What can I do now? And for how long? No one had answers to those all-important questions. We just had to wait and see. One more burden. The heaviness of "waiting". It had all grown to be just too much.

And one night, about ten years into this battle, in February of 2012, when I thought I could bear it no longer, I remember concluding that everyone's life would be better off without me. It just made perfect sense. Nobody would have to take care of me anymore, and as I couldn't even take care of my own family, what kind of mother did that make me? A failure. I felt like I was a failure at everything I had tried to build in my life. That was the heaviest burden of all to bear. On top of having just had yet another fight with my husband, I felt the very foundation of my life crumbling to dust beneath my feet. Or, more accurately, my wheels.

Yes. There was only one solution. One way to make things right… or at least as right as they could be. Take myself out of the equation.

So, I took my entire bottle of sleeping pills that night. I would solve my family's problems with one final sacrifice. I would be painless, for the first time in months even dare I say years. I would simply never wake up, and everyone else could breathe easier, knowing I wouldn't be a burden anymore. No more having to bathe me, care for my needs, or push me around in a wheelchair. They'd continue their lives, unburdened, and I would go and be with Jesus, for all eternity. Never again to hurt or be a burden to others.

As I waited for the sweet sleep to wash over me, I heard my six-year-old, Samuel, coming downstairs.

"Mommy!" he said as he threw his little boy arms around my neck. "I forgot to give you a hug and kiss goodnight!"

It hit me like a ton of bricks. "What in the hell did I just do!?"

That was the last thing I remember until I woke up two days later in the Intensive Care Unit of our local hospital. I can remember coming around, my eyes heavy-lidded, and thinking, "what happened? How did I get here?"

Soon, the flashbacks of that night came to me, along with a sense of elation that I was still alive. The realization that suicide was not the answer to my problems. It never had been, and never would be. I was incredibly grateful to God for sparing my life, yet still questioning, "Why?"

"Why keep me here while my family struggles to take care of me?" I cannot begin to explain the sense of helplessness, worthlessness that I felt because of this dastardly MS.

Before I was discharged from the hospital, a psychologist came to see me, just randomly assigned to my case. When he came in and sat down, literally the first words out of his mouth were, "what the hell were you thinking?"

I cried out my frustrations, my fears, my inadequacies. "I have no idea. I can assure you, in my right mind, I would NEVER have done this to my family. But, some days, I just feel like they'd be better off without me, because of my disease."

As he studied the list of the medications I had been taking, he shared, "do you realize the number one side effect of your MS med is suicide?"

NO! I had no idea!

He explained that he would prescribe antidepressants, to help counteract the tendency toward suicidal thinking that was accompanying my medication… and the hopelessness of my condition. I had already had antidepressants in the cocktail of daily meds I'd been taking, but it was clearly not enough. But, at the same time, he explained that he encouraged me to continue the MS med because my body needed it.

The reality of my condition began to hit me. "I am not going to be taking this medicine for the rest of my life. I don't know how, but this just isn't the answer."

A few days later, I was discharged from the hospital and returned home to begin my journey toward healing. One day, by the Grace of God, I came across a video posted to YouTube by a doctor named Terry Wahls. She had also been diagnosed with MS. She used a zero-gravity wheelchair yet was now riding her bike in marathons! This woman's story was nothing less than amazing!

I remember thinking, what did she do? How can she function like that if she has MS? I knew I simply had to dig deep, and not stop until I had the answers. If she could accomplish this… I could, too. I had to believe it! Deep in my soul.

Thus, in 2012 I began my Journey to Wellness. I would sit at my desk each day with my feet propped up on it, chair reclined, and a travel pillow placed backward under my neck, to allow me to hold my head up to be able to study the incredible story of Dr. Terry Wahls. I watched her videos and ordered the book she'd written of her own journey. I dug as deeply as I could to learn about the program she'd developed that allowed her to LIVE WITH MS, and not simply be DYING OF it.

Now, to be honest, I did not follow her program completely, but I was determined to take my life back, regardless, as she had. I would not be a victim of this disease, living a life of pain, misery, and disability. After all, I was only in my thirties, for cryin' out loud! I had five kids who needed me, and I needed to be whole again, for them as well as myself. I was fiercely and single-mindedly focused. I wasn't merely going to survive; I was going to LIVE.

My transformation from sickness to health began with a solid game plan and goals to be achieved. I decided one of the first goals in my new health care regimen would be to completely remove all the medications I'd been taking to treat my condition. I was excited, the day of my Neurologist's appointment, to tell him of my determination to take better control of my health, and to start from scratch. To go off all the meds that had been prescribed, and to follow the program Dr. Wahls had, to bring myself back to that measure of health she had accomplished. I would follow a healthier diet, supplement with vitamins and minerals that my body was likely lacking and see if I would find the improvement Dr. Wahls had. I asked my Neurologist for his help and support as I weaned myself from the unnatural drugs and followed this different path to healing. If this was possible, it was my intent.

My Neurologist's exact words to me were, "if you want to end up in a wheelchair, permanently, in less than five years, you go right ahead and give it a try. But you no longer need to come and see me, because I won't help you do that."

Just like that, my health journey of "we" became a path forward of "me." I would be charting my own course through the hurricane that my life had become. But I was ready. I just knew that I had found an avenue worth exploring, and I was all in. I never returned to that Neurologist again.

Day One, I discontinued taking all my prescribed meds. I quit all twelve of them cold turkey. Now, I don't recommend anyone working a health care regimen do that, but as I was now the captain and crew of my own ship, that was the decision I made, for me. I would no longer be tethered to a wheelchair; I was going to get my energy back. Be the mom I was destined to be and live my life as God designed it. And it wasn't going to be as an MS patient. My health care regimen would include anything, and everything involved with disease prevention. But pharmaceutical drugs, that merely masked symptoms and gave me awful side effects, had no part in that for me.

Something would be needed to replace those drugs. Food. Food became my medicine. It made complete sense. I revamped my entire diet, and went 100% raw, which meant eating nothing but fresh, uncooked fruits and vegetables, sprouted nuts, seeds, and grains. It is not the diet that everyone may need to repair their bodies, but it turned out to be the answer for me.

I remember my mother coming to the house and helping me prep my food. We'd sit at the kitchen table together, chopping fruits and vegetables. I could barely hold my head up, I was so weak and tired, so I would lay my upper body across the table for support and chop the food while lying sideways. I remember my mom making me a homemade juice to try and replenish my energy, and

I drank it readily, convinced that God made food to nourish and heal our bodies and that if I used food the way He intended, He would heal me.

It wasn't long before I started seeing the results…literally… for which I'd prayed, so long.

Within three weeks of having begun my new eating plan, I regained 20/20 vision in my right eye. I had made such progress that I went from complete blindness in that eye, to having perfect vision! Outside of eliminating the prescription drugs, the only thing that had changed was the foods I chose to eat. Three weeks after that, I was able to take our dog for a walk for the first time in nearly eleven years. And within nine weeks from the start of my Healthcare Journey, I was symptom free.

That is what eating the proper foods, in their most basic form, did for my body. My mind. And my health. (My case is rare, not the norm. But I hope it encourages you as to what is possible.)

Now did it put my MS into complete remission? Was I cured of Chronic Fatigue Syndrome and Fibromyalgia? I can't say that. What I CAN say is that I fed my body the nutrients and live enzymes it needed. I filled myself with the minerals and vitamins my immune system used to restore my health and get me to a place where my own body could combat those conditions. And, just as I had experienced when I was pregnant with Samuel, my symptoms went away, completely. Whatever had been attacking me was gone. Eliminated, or driven dormant, once again. This time, not to return. And I don't anticipate ever putting myself into such a state of physical dysfunction again.

I've learned quite a bit along the way, as I embarked on this Journey and struggled to regain my health. Much of what I learned has led me along a path away from Allopathic Medicine… the standard practice of medicine utilized by most classically trained MDs. While Allopathic Medicine does have its place in the practice of Health Care, it is not the only way that an optimum state of Health is achieved. Some might argue it is rarely the way. As the focus of Allopathic Medicine seems to have evolved, in many doctor's practices, into a matter of "diagnose and treat disease states", as opposed to a goal of achieving and maintaining wellness, many patients who rely solely on Allopathic Medicine don't bother to visit their doctors until they are feeling so ill that the concept of "health" is absent in their lives.

In my quest for optimal health, I've had to change my mindset in numerous fashions.

One conclusion I have reached, from my studies, as well as my personal health journey, is that I do not believe in "autoimmune disease" in the classic sense. Although I acknowledge the existence of genetic diseases, that is a topic for another chapter… and another day. But typically, we are told by Health Care Practitioners that an autoimmune disease is the result of our body just randomly starting to attack our organs and causing them to malfunction, without recognizable cause in many cases, and that the treatment for many of these incurable conditions is a lifetime of pharmaceutical drugs.

My studies have led me to believe that, in the instance of most "disease" some situations trigger the body to not function properly. Such as the "invasion" by a pathogen. The body's response to the intruder is to attempt to stop the damage being caused as the offender grows, reproduces, and harms various systems of the body and to do that, it reacts to its environment, putting out "danger signals" we interpret as "symptoms." Our bodies use whatever "weapons" they have in their arsenal to attack the "invaders" … be they of a bacterial, viral, parasitic, fungal, mold, toxic chemical, or heavy metal origin. For example, if the body has been overtaken by a bacterium, reproducing faster than the body is prepared to fight, and the immune system hasn't enough weaponry to fight them off, it cannot win the battle, and the invading pathogen starts to wreak havoc within bodily systems. Left to its own devices, the enemy will win the war.

In my own case, my body responded to the various returns of my EBV by attacking the protective coating of the nerves throughout my body, the myelin sheaths, and disrupting the messages being sent back and forth from my brain to my muscles, and vice versa. Soon, my body could no longer act on what the brain was telling it to do, and a complete breakdown of my body's abilities was the result. The medicines my doctor prescribed did not solve the problem because, although they were designed to treat the symptoms, they did not address the root cause of the problem to begin with.

My mother was diagnosed with Alzheimer's Disease. The brains of Alzheimer's sufferers develop "amyloid plaque", a sort of collection of proteins and cellular debris, that coat different parts of the brain, and are thought to bring about the effects of sometimes decades of accumulation of toxic chemicals, hormonal imbalances, and/or heavy metals, further damaging the brain's cells and preventing their proper functioning. The side effects of this "amyloid cloud" that infuses the brain result in memory loss and a gradual lessening of bodily awareness and functioning. But this is not a problem caused by the body attacking itself. The body was attempting to stop the invasion and build-up of whatever was poisoning the brain in the first place.

That is what takes place within the body of those suffering from "autoimmune diseases."

The more I learned about the cause of "disease" and the body's ability and desire to heal itself if presented with the proper tools… the more I felt a calling to learn more. And to be able to not only restore my own body's ability to function at its peak, but to learn how to help others as well. I didn't feel it was enough to simply have resolved my own health disruption, I needed more in-depth study and understanding of Health, and how to achieve and retain it, in order to truly feel I was prepared to counsel and assist others.

So, my journey broadened, and intensified. In 2014, my Husband and I divorced, and I continued my journey to health as a single mom, for the next five years. In 2015 I enrolled in a two-year course of study offered through the Institute of Integrative Nutrition, with the goal to become a Nutrition and Health Coach. Two years after completing these studies, my Certificate as a Health Coach securely in hand, I began coursework to obtain my Doctorate in Functional Medicine at the School of Applied Functional Medicine (SAFM). I worked at this approach for a year and a half, at which time, I was introduced to a Wholistic Health Care Practitioner who incorporated biofeedback, through the use of Electrodermal Screening (EDS) into her practice. For those who may never have heard of EDS, it is a manner of using a computer-based program to measure and assess the flow of electrical current through every body system and organ (biofeedback). Much as an EKG (electrocardiogram) assesses the electrical functioning of the heart, or an EEG (electroencephalogram) can be used to determine proper electrical function within the brain, EDS measures the electrical activity and health of body organs and systems, assessing for malfunctions and inadequacies that lead to conditions we typically refer to as "disease." As I had learned in my Functional Medicine studies, it is necessary to do a "root cause analysis" ... to search for malfunctions within the "root" of the human system that are the basis of a person's illness, and to repair these breakdowns, thereby "fixing the problem," not merely applying pharmaceutical drugs to the symptoms, much like salve and a Band-Aid. This approach, along with other similarly focused tools, truly leads to "Health Care" and not just "illness treatment."

When scanned by the EDS system, I learned I had a "four prong" root cause of my body's dis-ease, as well as my MS symptoms. Not only was the EBV found, as I'd already known, but also fluoride toxicity, (likely from decades of drinking fluoridated water and brushing my teeth daily with fluoridated toothpaste. [In case you weren't aware, fluoride is a neurotoxin]) heavy metal toxicity, primarily silver amalgam, (the composition of cavity fillings common in dental practices of my youth) and a spirochete bacterium in my spinal cord and throughout my nervous system. As well as numerous pesticides, insecticides, and fungicides that had built up over years of breathing in these toxins, as well as consuming them in commercially grown fruits and vegetables. With the EDS analysis, it was revealed that, when the four main factors were removed from the scan results, my body showed no signs or symptoms of MS, but when the EBV, fluoride, silver, and the spirochete were factored back in, my Multiple Sclerosis symptoms registered. Once I had cleared my system of these four factors, including having all my silver fillings removed by a biological dentist, specially trained in the safe removal of amalgam fillings,** and replaced with toxin-free fillings, my body healed itself of the MS signs and symptoms, and repaired the myelin sheath, allowing me to regain full function of my body. I learned firsthand what a valuable tool EDS could be in the practice of Functional Medicine.

As I grew to more fully understand the purpose and practice of EDS, I wished to become more fluent and able to incorporate this new tool into my own ongoing personal maintenance and, someday, into my ability to counsel and lead others to their own improved states of health. I was soon working side by side with my new mentor, learning from her as well as the doctors, instructors, and other practitioners who had helped her learn and grow throughout her thirty-year-long career. I was impressed at discovering how many patients were being treated, and the distance from which so many traveled, simply to have access to the EDS technology and its health benefits.

At the same time, I continued my studies by shifting my focus from obtaining a Functional Medicine degree, instead, toward my Doctorate in Naturopathy, allowing me to not only counsel others to improved health through the identification of the root causes of their illnesses and restoration of proper body functioning, but to be able to utilize EDS to test, and to prescribe the homeopathic remedies, as well as the supplements and vitamins that work to restore proper immune function. I am currently working through the Doctor of Naturopathy program at the School of Energetic Wellness. I am hoping to be board certified by the end of 2023.

I have also completed coursework to be a Certified Functional Bloodwork Specialist and have been utilizing this tool in my practice. With this additional certification, I can analyze blood work ordered, drawn and assessed at labs throughout the U.S. and factor these results into my patients' care and treatment needs. Therefore, utilizing these results to help people go from unhealthy to healthy regardless of their symptoms or diagnosis.

My Health Care and Coaching practice currently helps people who suffer from various health conditions and have been to doctors, specialists, had all the labs drawn and tests run but just aren't getting healthier, I'm here to tell you there is an alternative way to better health! I work with people who deal with chronic colds/flu to different "autoimmune" issues and even chronic illnesses and diseases. My goal isn't to heal or cure you, but to make you healthy again and get you back to living and enjoying life!!!

My practice involves some of the following modalities or can include them all. Blood work analysis, EDS screening, dietary planning and management, colonic bowel cleansing, lymphatic drainage therapy, foot detox baths, root cause analysis of your disease as well as the utilization of homeopathic remedies and food grade supplements of vitamins and minerals in an individualized health care plan. I can schedule both virtual or in person visits regardless of your location, as my current practice routinely schedules in person visits with clients traveling from New York to California and most states in between. For that I am humbled and grateful. Please note that virtual visits will limit the healing modalities we use but are still beneficial and many clients are utilizing the virtual visit technology today.

So back to my original question...

"How did I get here?"

If "here" is my now optimal state of health, I'd say I got here by determination, willpower, and the Grace of God.

But more specifically, I changed my diet. I know that's not very clear. If I were to give general dietary advice, I would say EAT Clean, Whole Foods above all. My rule is if Man made it, don't eat it!! If God made it, ENJOY. Please do NOT eat or consume any oils other than these...Extra Virgin Olive Oil or as Rachel Ray says "EVOO," Avocado Oil, Real Butter, Coconut Oil (Unrefined-Tastes like coconut, Refined-Flavorless), Lard or Tallow. Any other oil will be inflammatory!!! Especially avoid Vegetable Oil, Canola Oil or any other man-made oil. Surprisingly, sunflower seed oil and most seed oils are inflammatory as well. This makes eating out a challenge. However, I tell the server I have an allergy to oils and ask what oils they use or say, "I can only have olive oil or real butter" and they usually assist me with the menu. Always read ingredients and follow this rule for reducing inflammation and improving your health.

As I changed my diet, and began to reduce inflammation and pain, my brain became clearer and less muddled. My mindset shifted. It was now easier to declare, "I will take my life back. I will get healthy and have more energy. I will walk without assistance."

I went from "I can't" to "I will!" I really focused on my mindset and worked on thinking positively. And I am here to tell you, the more you tell yourself positive things, the more you start to believe them. The mind is a powerful tool.

My family and friends were key in my healing process. They were my support system, encouraging and helpful when I needed it. Tough and demanding when THAT was the kick in the pants that got me going. I urge you to ask for help if needed. And accept it, when offered. I am the first to say, "I know it's not easy!!" But it was what I needed, and I believe from the bottom of my heart, nobody makes it through the difficulties in life, especially health issues, alone! Find people who will help, support, and encourage you. Don't try to do it alone.

No matter what, even in the darkest times, look up! God is always there. I have asked God to allow me to curl up in his lap and hold me when I felt alone. As a matter of fact, there was a period, several years, where I was mad at God. I remember thinking, "if you're still there why are you letting me go through this? Where are you?" I was angry, feeling alone and abandoned by God.

Looking back, I can now see that I was never alone. He was always there. And this journey I traveled was needed to make me who I am today. To bring me through the things I went through to be able to help others who are suffering the way I did. All in all, I see God's grace, love and mercy on me as I traveled down some of the darkest roads.

He brought me to it; He brought me through it. And now I'm prepared to help you, my reader, to do the same.

Come, take my hand, and let's get started on YOUR Health Journey.

Visit www.wheelchair2walking.com to see the current programs I have available and to connect with me personally. I look forward to helping you take your life back, like I did.

— Kristie

Kristie Hess-Newton

https://www.facebook.com/hess.kristie

Visit my private group Body and Soul Nourishment for recipes and general health and wellness info. Please answer BOOK in Question of How did you hear about this group to be approved!

https://www.facebook.com/groups/166286530548406/

** If you would like to know if there is a dentist near you who can safely remove your toxic silver fillings go to https://iabdm.org or www.https://iaomt.org for a listing.

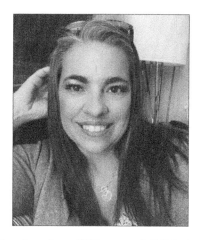

Kristie Hess-Newton is a Wife, as of 2019, to Greg Newton, Mother of five children, Hanna, Jacob, Jeremiah, Samuel and Sera, and Step-Mother to three more, Alicia, Alexis, and Isaiah, and Grandmother of five. She is passionate about helping others heal the mind, body and spirit through alternative health and therapeutic prayer ministry. She has used therapeutic prayer ministry for more than twenty-four years and gives all glory to God for any health and healing she and her clients experience.

CHAPTER 12:

The Relationship Between Gut and Hormones

By: Jessica Milner, MSHN, FBWS

I used to be the girl who was overweight, tired, and couldn't even drink chicken broth without having an Irritable Bowel Syndrome (IBS) attack. I was a completely different person. I was the one who was always looking for the bathroom, and had to know where it was. I was terrified of going on long car rides, or airplanes, or taking vacations at all because I needed to have all of these pharmaceutical medications with me to combat all of the things that were always hurting me. I was a walking pharmacy. Particularly, I would have IBS attacks all the time, and they were pretty unpredictable, it didn't seem to matter what I ate. As time went on, I started to gain weight uncontrollably, and then came to find out that I was dealing with infertility as well.

I had doctors telling me that my labs were absolutely fine yet my joints were killing me, my stomach was killing me, and no matter what fertility drugs they gave me, I wasn't getting pregnant. I had gastrointestinal (GI) doctors tell me that it didn't matter what I ate because my GI symptoms had nothing to do with eating. And I think that that was a pivotal moment for me because how could that possibly be? How can something that I'm putting into my digestive system not have anything to do with the pain I'm experiencing? That was just so weird. Going through years of fertility treatment with nothing but frustration was taxing on my body and relationships, and did not resolve until I started incorporating holistic and natural measures...the same ones the doctors told me would have no effect on my conditions.

Of course that's going over many years in a tiny little nutshell. But eventually I was able to figure out that certain foods, personal and household products, and emotions were playing a huge role in my stress, and helped me begin my holistic journey. After years of frustration, my husband and I were blessed with twin girls, and we now have two boys as well! On my journey to becoming a mom, I started with more little bits of holistic measures to get myself feeling better, this didn't happen overnight! It was years of small changes with big results and eventually I found myself in school for a master's in holistic nutrition, and then working clinically as a functional holistic nutritionist.

I often wish I had known back then what I know now, but we all have a journey for a reason I have now been able to realize a greater purpose to help others overcome these issues so they don't have to worry about missing out on an entire wedding reception or somebody's baby shower or the summer barbecue or whatever fun event they're attending because they end up spending the entire time in the bathroom instead. Those are no longer worries for me. I am now able to take long car rides without the anxiety of where the next rest stop is, I do not need an entire suitcase just for my medications, my cycles are a breeze most months, and my weight is well-managed. Ten years ago, I would have thought this impossible.

There's a huge connection between your gut and your hormones, it really should be talked about more. I mentioned that I had

THE RELATIONSHIP BETWEEN GUT AND HORMONES

problems with infertility and with weight management and those things are absolutely hormonal. Your gut has so much to do with those hormones. The connection is really underrated in our conventional system because they don't view the body as a whole system working together, they look at parts instead. We aren't cars, yo. We are way more than just the sum of our parts.

Your gut needs to have the correct permeability in order for your hormones to properly be produced and send the proper signals. Okay, what does that mean? You want your gut lining to keep things in that should be in, and things out that should be out. Your hormones need to be balanced in order for your gut to be healthy, so it really works both ways. You have your gut-brain axis, and hormones are crucial for your gut-brain axis. You have things like leaky gut, IBS, Crohn's, and these are all linked with hormone disorders. Even hormones like ghrelin, which regulates hunger, and leptin, which regulates your satiety. If these hormones are out of balance, you might never feel hungry, or you might just always be hungry and just want to eat all the things. When you have chronic inflammation of the gut, inflammation molecules mess with the proper function of hormones and the pathways they take. So this is going to lead to things like insulin resistance, Polycystic Ovarian Syndrome (PCOS) and thyroid imbalances. These are some things that I was experiencing. And these are a lot of the things that people who come to see me now have been experiencing….and yet their labs look "fine."

It's interesting how much your gut is influenced by estrogen & progesterone. If they are imbalanced, you can totally experience gut issues like bloating, constipation, and diarrhea. If you have back and forth constipation to diarrhea, it's likely that you have some imbalances with your progesterone and estrogen going on. Based on this, someone should have known much sooner based on my GI symptoms that these hormones were suffering.

Stress is another huge factor in hormones and gut health. Stress triggers stress hormones like cortisol, and when you have chronically elevated cortisol, it really damages your gut permeability and your microbiota. This is going to lead to leaky gut and other hormones will absolutely tank.

Stress is pretty much unavoidable, but your emotional and traumatic side of healing is absolutely important. It's important that you cleanse your energetic vital body as well as work on your physical body. The energy that surrounds us actually holds all of the blueprints for your physical body, so if it's not healthy, then your physical body is never going to totally be healthy. I offer an energy work modality called Body Code to help address those traumatic and emotional sides to healing. So that is something that is a little bit unique in my programs, I always make sure that that area of healing is being addressed because sometimes it's the very wall blocking someone's pathway to feeling better.

My background is in nutrition so a lot of people are intimidated by that. But all I want from you is to eat real food. There are some inflammatory foods that may need to be avoided for a time like grains and dairy, but in the end I want to see you eating real food. Ultra-processed food is usually full of additives, chemicals used in conventional farming, and rancid seed oils. These things will tax your liver, remove and block minerals, decrease hormone production, cause mega-inflammation, and do a number on your gut. So focusing on real food and keeping sugar to a bare minimum is my best advice for that. This also helps you burn fat for fuel, which will help keep your hormones and weight in check. There is no need to name your diet. Just be human and eat real food.

I like to design clinical protocols based on the individual. My protocols are usually similar for many patients, but everybody's imbalances are going to be different. We're going to want to tackle the imbalances of the gut based on what your gut actually needs.

I'm talking about toxicity here, we all have it. The difference is *the stressor* causing the toxicity. For years, applied kinesiology has been a major part of my work and I love it because I can identify stressors by using your body's own reflexes, and digging into lab work really opens it up even more. We can determine based on your regular labs that your doctor insists are completely normal…because they do have answers in them that can tell us what types of support your body needs. What organs need support? Are you utilizing your nutrients properly? Your labs have these answers and we can use them to design a program to tackle your specific needs…so you can start feeling better, like yourself again, and not care where the bathroom is. So you don't need to wonder why even though you've been going to the gym every single day and watching what you eat you've gained thirty pounds of fat! Things that are super frustrating because no matter what you do as far as eating healthy and exercising, you're still feeling gross. We don't want to feel sick, we don't want to feel gross, we don't want to wonder where the bathroom is, we don't want to be in pain all of the time, or even most of the time!

People who come to see me usually have issues with digestion, annoying weight gain, painful or irregular periods, or they're starting perimenopause/menopause…but I get folks with skin issues and allergies a lot too. Most have "normal" labs and no actual answers to their pain and are coming to me as a last resort. I honestly love being the last practitioner they need to see before feeling better!

I had one woman who was experiencing such pain with her periods that she would be in bed for days and even vomit from the pain. Within three cycles, we had her able to go about her day during her period. The first month, she was in bed but did not vomit from the pain. The second month, she was in pain but not stuck in bed. The third month, she couldn't believe she was able to leave the house and go to work during her period. After years of suffering each month, there was much rejoicing!

I had another woman come to me who would only have a bowel movement once every six days on average. Her longest was twenty-four days!! She felt awful, her body was toxic, she was overweight and always uncomfortable. Over the next two months, we were able to get her bowels moving everyday and she would almost dance into my office for follow-ups! She was a new woman not just because she was able to go to the bathroom, but because the toxicity that was stuck inside her was addressed and she was no longer being controlled by the bad bacteria & fungi that had been in charge for so long. Her pants fit better and she is absolutely glowing now.

I get a wide variety of people but their issues stem down to gut and hormone health. Most of us are walking around with toxicity we can't see and we are wondering why we feel the way we do. The truth is: every illness whether chronic or acute, every organ dysfunction, every nutrient deficiency stems from some kind of toxicity. My job is to find the toxicity, remove it, and support the body so you can start feeling better. This is my passion. I lived through it myself, I get it, and as a result, I will listen and empathize. I know how imperative it is for you to have results. This is your life, and you need to take it back so you can live it!

If you want to follow me for tips, recipes, mom life and my silliness, you can find me on Facebook at Deep Rooted Wellness! https://www.facebook.com/deeprootedwellnessid/

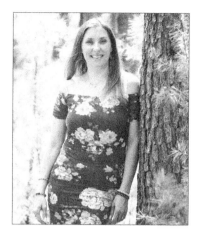

Jessica Milner, MSHN, FBWS is a clinical nutritionist and functional bloodwork specialist. Jess earned an Associate's degree from The Restaurant School at Walnut Hill College and a BS from Saint Joseph's University before achieving her Master's degree in Holistic Nutrition, with Honors, from American College of Healthcare Sciences. She is also a Certified Body Code Practitioner. Jess lives in North Idaho with her husband and their four children, two dogs, and a turtle. When she is not working, you can find her dancing in her kitchen, laughing with her husband, hiking, studying, lifting some weights, crushing a Buti yoga class, snuggling her pit bulls, or homeschooling her kiddos.

CHAPTER 13:
Western and Eastern Medicine

By: Tracy Chambers

Have you ever gone to the doctor feeling crummy only to be told that your labs are "normal" and that there's nothing wrong with you? As a Functional Blood Work Specialist, I know that there is nothing more defeating or disheartening than feeling bad, being told everything is "fine," and having no clear direction on how to get better and feel like yourself again. I am honored to help my patients address the pain under the pain, and I am proud of the journey that brought me here.

I started my own journey to find and promote holistic wellness as a Fitness and Nutrition

Specialist, and later became a licensed Massage Therapist and Personal Trainer. To supplement this practice, I earned my Master's in Acupuncture, and later became a Registered

Nurse. This combination of Eastern and Western medicine practices allows me to get to the bottom of my patients' pain points because I am able to peel back the different layers that contribute to an overall feeling of un-wellness. Having this variety of tools in my toolbox has enabled me to look at various issues through different lenses to find the missing pieces of the puzzle in order to see the full picture and empower my patients to heal. While our bodies are amazing, we must nurture them and identify and clear out the physical, mental, emotional, or spiritual blocks that prevent us from reaching our full potential.

Throughout the course of our lives, we will all encounter factors that challenge our bodies' state of balance and lead to disease. In order to be truly healthy, we must be well in five areas: physical, mental, emotional, spiritual, and energy. If one aspect is out of order, our bodies compensate to keep the other systems functioning, which, over time, can cause physical symptoms. Though unpleasant to experience, symptoms are guideposts that can provide us with insight as to what is off balance and help us determine what steps we need to take to get back to a balanced state. In my practice, I have learned to identify and address the early symptoms and help my patients address the problems before they turn into full-scale crises. In today's world of information overload, I often see clients who are doing "all the right things," but still just don't feel good. When you feel like you have tried everything, I can help you determine what will actually work for you and your unique situation.

Growing up, I loved being outdoors, spending time in the woods, visiting the beach, and being barefoot. I was also a competitive athlete and poured my energy into competitive sports. In the midst of treks through the woods, visits to the beach, sports tournaments, and your typical high school drama, I was also diagnosed with Mono three separate times in four years. My doctor found it odd, as my adrenals and thyroid were always in the "normal" range. I would later learn that, once contracted, the EBV virus remains dormant in the body and can "flare up" when provoked. Refusing to accept the doctor's insistence that everything was "fine," my mom took me to specialists who were practicing functional medicine even before the field was officially established.

These specialists worked on healing my gut, supporting my adrenals and thyroid, and added B vitamin supplements to my diet to alter my energy pathways. Of course, being young and not knowing any differently, once I started feeling better, I dropped the strategies that were helping me to feel better. Initially, this was fine, but before long, my body started screaming at me again.

Both my passion for sports and my interest in nutrition inspired me to major in Nutrition and Exercise. When recovering from an injury, I underwent massage therapy, which led me to become a licensed Massage Therapist. In an effort to prevent future injuries and practice functional fitness, I also earned multiple certifications in Personal Training, Strength Training, Conditioning, Medical Massage Therapy, and Post Rehab Strength and Conditioning. Even before graduating from college, I opened up a private Massage Therapy and Personal Training Practice.

Despite my successes, I hit another period in my early twenties where I just felt terrible all the time. I was depressed and had very low energy. I started working with another woman who addressed my issues layer by layer, starting with my blood work. Again, my body needed some of the same support—adrenals, thyroid, gut support, vitamins, and minerals—as it did when I was recovering from Mono. I also worked with a woman who offered IV nutritional therapy. As I began to feel better, I realized that my body was susceptible to the same patterns of dysfunction if I didn't care for it properly, and I also came to understand that it would require different strategies during different times of the year in order to optimally function at the cellular level.

As my own health improved, my practice grew, and it felt great to help my clients achieve their health goals. However, something was missing, and I was very aware of the scope of my practice and its limitations. I had always been intrigued when I worked with functional medicine practitioners, but I didn't know what steps to take to gain that skill, and life had a different plan. I still wanted to expand my scope, provide a more holistic model of healing, and be able to better help my clients. So, I went back to school and earned my Master's in Acupuncture, which also introduced me to the world of Eastern medicine and enabled me to better shape my practice.

During this time in my career, I married, had children, and got divorced. As a single mom of three littles, I needed a stable income and a more structured work schedule, I went back to school to become a registered nurse. While I learned a great deal that I knew would help me help my patients, I became very aware of the broken healthcare system in the United States. I found working as an RN to be incredibly limited after having my own practice. I grew increasingly discouraged with the American healthcare system, disillusioned with Western medicine's sole focus on treating only the symptoms of disease, and frustrated by my own restricted role in helping my patients regain their health so that they could once again fully participate in their active lives.

As my children got older, I was able to dive into what really intrigued me: Functional Blood work, and using the labs my clients already had to find the missing pieces of the puzzle in order to help them. Combining my knowledge, experience, and understanding of the human body with the best parts of both Western and Eastern medicine has empowered me to individually and holistically address patient needs in order to enable them to heal and feel their best.

I am very passionate about working with women and girls to help them reclaim their energy and live their lives to the fullest. For example, I have worked with many women with menopausal symptoms who have been told by the doctor that their labs are normal, even though they are experiencing a long list of symptoms that prevent them from going about their daily lives. I am able to identify and address the causes of the symptoms and help these women feel like themselves again. In addition, I am always excited to work with girls aged thirteen to twenty to address their chronic fatigue and enable them to expend their energy on spending time with friends and succeeding in school instead of being stuck in bed with no clear path on how to feel better.

One of my clients is, like me, a mom with three kids. When she first started seeing me, she felt depressed, and spent days laying in bed, feeling guilty that she wasn't able to be there for her kids. She dealt with weight gain, acid reflux, chronic fatigue, insomnia, hot flashes, and painful periods that eventually led to a hysterectomy. After reviewing her blood work, I was able to identify where there were deficiencies that needed to be supported, which areas needed to be healed, which cofactors needed to be added, and what aspects of the brain chemistry could be altered to aid in good sleep. In short, I was able to give her body the building blocks needed to promote the innate power of the body to heal itself. Receiving a call from her saying that she was sleeping well at night, alert, in less pain, and most importantly, able to be present for her family was one of the proudest moments of my career.

The more I expand my practice and learn about different modalities, the better I am able to effectively utilize both Western and Eastern medicine. As I grow as a practitioner, my ultimate goal remains the same: I want to work with those that are told their lab work is normal but still feel bad or unwell so that they can live healthy and fulfilling lives. Our bodies are wise and constantly give us signals about what they need, but society and our fast-paced culture have created a disconnect within our bodies that makes it difficult to always identify and act on these signals. We are spread thin in life and our bodies need support. While we can't always change or eliminate stressors entirely, I can use lab work to identify, decrease, and manage internal stressors. I am here to support you, make sure your body has what it needs to care for itself. I believe that it is best to speak to the pain under the pain to help you reclaim health and joy in your life.

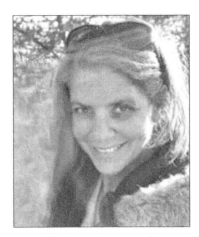

Tracy lives in Annapolis, Maryland, and has three young-adult children. She offers a Virtual Practice to help clients who are struggling with their health, even though they have been told that their labs are normal. Tracy helps patients identify the hidden pieces of the puzzle contributing to their health issues in order to help those feeling unhealthy to feel healthy again.

Through her practice, Tracy empowers clients to feel like themselves again. Growing up, Tracy was an outdoorsy girl who loved spending time at the beach, and she was also active in competitive sports. In college, she earned degrees in Fitness and Nutrition and Small Business Management. She is also a massage therapist, and in 1994 she opened her practice: Enhance Your Health, Inc., which offers Personal Training, Massage Therapy, and Nutritional Coaching.

Over time, she wanted to fill in what she felt were treatment gaps, so she added both Western and Eastern Medicine to her arsenal by becoming a Registered Nurse and receiving her

Master's Degree in Acupuncture. Later on, she earned an additional certification as a Functional Blood Work Specialist. In her current practice, Tracy uses all the tools in her toolbox to help identify what is causing the feelings of dis-ease in her clients and uses effective interventions to support their bodies and help them feel healthy. If you are ready to take control of your health, email Tracy at enhanceyourhealthnow@gmail.com.

CHAPTER 14:

Case Study: Andrea, Age 52

By: Dina Rabo, DC

Do you, or someone you know, have a list of symptoms like Andrea?

- Chronic pain
- Anxiety
- Depression
- Panic attacks
- Brain fog
- Muscle weakness
- Daily fatigue
- Low energy
- Sleep apnea
- Can't get out of bed in the morning
- Joint pain
- Low libido
- Hair thinning
- Allergies
- Frequent colds and flu

Does your life sound like hers?

- Busy and stressful
- Usually puts herself last
- Struggling to make it through each day
- So many tests and lots of doctors, with NO answers
- Feeling like she's not being heard
- On many medications or supplements
- Relationships are suffering
- Surgery or other drastic measures are on the horizon

So, what do you do about all this? Seems overwhelming! But it's simple.

For Andrea, Dr. Dina Rabo looked for the "hidden weaknesses" in her regular blood work (No special tests required).

From the blood work, she found:

- Hormone dysregulation
- Blood sugar imbalances
- Inflammation
- Low iron
- Low vitamin D
- Autoimmune indicators
- Chronic low grade viral infection
- Adrenal fatigue

The answers inside the test results helped her create a course of action to give Andrea's body the right environment to start healing itself.

The game plan:

- Reduce the stress inside her body
- Eliminate inflammation

- Balance blood sugar
- Support her adrenals
- Rebuild and support her gut
- Boost immune system
- All of the above automatically help in resolving hormone issues

All with diet, supplements, awareness, rebalancing microbiome and stress reduction.

Four months later, Andrea is making great progress!
- Lowered anti depression medication
- Much less anxiety
- More energy
- Enjoying her work
- Significant decrease in pain
- Able to exercise
- Has become more aware of when things are off in her body

Three Takeaways:
1. Find the hidden weaknesses in your blood work—work to get levels to their *optimal* ranges.
2. Reduce internal stressors—then the body can handle the external stressors much better.
3. Learn to listen to your own body so you can take care of yourself before things get too bad (put your own oxygen mask on before helping others put theirs on!)

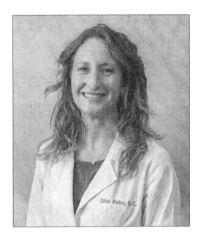

Dina Rabo-Alexander is a chiropractor and health coach of Rabo Health and Wellness in Chico California. She specializes in whole body wellness, utilizing chiropractic technique, functional bloodwork, and the latest in regenerative therapy, including non-invasive stem cell treatment and infrared light therapy to help the body heal at a cellular level. You may go to RaboChiropracticCenter.com or find her on Instagram at RaboHealth.com.

CHAPTER 15:

Four Quick Strategies to Improve Gut Function

By: James E. Hicks, DC, CFMP

*L*earn the Four Quick Strategies to Improve Gut Function so that you can have great looking skin resounding with beauty and radiance!

Are you a busy working mom, multi-tasking, to get it all done in a day? Need more hours in the day? Do you suffer from problematic skin? Are you starting to feel or look older than what you think you ought to be? Is your fast-lane lifestyle of chronic stress, poor food choices, exposure to over-bounding toxicity in your foods, water, air, home, workplace, personal body care products, kitchenware, cosmetics, soaps, detergents you use, the blame for problematic skin problems like eczema or acne that may be the culprits that are causing digestive issues like Leaky Gut or Irritable Bowel Syndrome?

1. The Importance of Creating a Healthy Home...
You Can't Have Beautiful Skin If Your Home Isn't Healthy

If you want to get well, stay well, and have beautiful looking skin, you may need to consider implementing the following strategies that may significantly improve your overall health issues as a starting point:

1) Reduce exposure to your home and office EMFs (Electro Magnetic Fields)

Mitigation may include the following measures:
- Minimize cell phone use.
- Minimize your use of portable phones at home and shift to a corded phone.
- Rent or purchase a meter to test for EMFs in your home (EMFcenter.com).
- Hardwire your computer and TV so that you can turn off your wifi via ethernet.
- Consider putting a kill switch or timer device to shut off the wifi before going to bed.
- Use the speaker device as much as practical on your phone instead of placing it on your ear.
- Do not place your laptop on your lap.
- Do not sleep in the same room as your router.
- Take the clock radio away from the head of your bed.
- Unplug your router at night.
- See if you can opt-out of a smart meter on your home/property. Otherwise, protect yourself from these smart meters (SmartMeterGuard.com).
- Get the fields measured in a potential new car before you buy it. (www.ewg.org).

2) Minimize Blue Light
- Wear blue blocker glasses when using cell phones, tablets and TV at night when the sun goes down.
- As long as light hits the eye, the brain perceives that it is still daylight, prolonging melatonin to kick in for deep restful sleep. Blue blocker glasses help mitigate that concern. Restful deep sleep is vital to the repair and restore process of the body while sleeping.

3) Household and Cleaning Products
- Minimize and/or avoid the use of chemicals on the skin such as commercial lotions, creams, colognes, perfumes, soaps, deodorants, laundry detergent, shampoos, conditioners, body washes, make-up, hair coloring, cosmetics, lipsticks. www.primallifeorganics.com
- Natural make-up sold at Whole Foods, 100% pure. www.100percentpure.com
- Personal care products: https://www.ewg.org/skindeep/
- Avoid hairspray, nail polish, perfumes (use essential oils), aluminum based antiperspirants, products containing synthetic fragrances, hair products (including shampoo and colors) with alcohol, sodium lauryl sulfate, paraben, phthalate or other petrochemicals, toothpaste with fluoride in it.
- Search for organic products from Whole Foods, Trader Joe's, Amazon, Young Living.
- Use vinegar for surface cleaning or with laundry.
- Refrain from using plastic containers. Switch to glass like Mason Jars.
- Use stainless steel or ceramic cast iron cookware. Avoid teflon and aluminum cookware.
- Wear natural clothing: cotton, silk, or wool. Avoid polyester.
- Use bamboo toilet paper or versus recycle. Avoid BPA in toilet paper and paper towels.
- Credit card receipts are toxic. Request a text receipt where practical.
- Use a wool or bamboo mattress topper or 100% latex mattress to protect from the flame retardants.
- Use organic sheets.

4) Mold
- Test for mold. If you live in a house that has mold, and has not been remediated, you may have the most difficult time to get healthy, stay healthy, and have beautiful skin.
- Standing water, water leaks, wet drywall, laundry front-end loader washers that leak water from the door hatch are all a foundation for mold growth.
- Antique furniture, attics, basements, old musty books/magazines become a concern for mold.

5) Dental
- Your digestion and health starts in your mouth. Each tooth corresponds to an organ structure. A dysfunctional tooth may correlate and be predictive of a health issue in the body. Refer to the attached Meridian Tooth Chart below:

Meridian Tooth Chart

- Choose your dentist wisely. Why is this important? Conventional dentists are still using mercury (silver amalgams) to apply to cavities and are convinced that if it

is sealed in the tooth, that it is safe. Mercury is a very harmful substance to the body and brain. This heavy metal may wreak havoc on your ability to heal, let alone having radiant unblemished skin.
- Consider seeking the help of a biological dentist in the future. Biological dentistry focus is that dental and oral health is fundamentally connected to a patient's overall health and they use minimally invasive procedures with biocompatible materials.
- The International Academy of Oral Medicine and Toxicology (IAOMT) certified dentists are the ones to seek out for optimal preservation of oral health.

2. Proper Diet & Hydration

The plan of having beautiful radiant skin, one must initially look at the diet, first and foremost. We need to find the "sweet spot" for the diet that is energetically compatible with your make-up. You have to recognize that you have an outer skin and an inner skin (gut lining from your mouth to your anus). When you lose the integrity of the one cell membrane in your gut, the result can be any host of many bodily problems, to include all types of problematic skin.

Secondly, we need to minimize and eliminate our exposure to toxins (in the air, food, environment, viruses, bacteria, fungus, yeast, mold, heavy metals, parasites) that wreak havoc on the permeable gut lining affecting the microbiome. When you experience eczema, dermatitis, psoriasis, or acne, you try to hide the outward expression of those conditions. Bad looking skin can be a stigma that wreaks havoc on your self-esteem and confidence in the presence of others in public. With all the stress in your life, sometimes you just don't have the time to properly take care of yourself through your diet. So what you typically do in most cases, is resort to applying make-up, lotions, creams, moisturizes, resorting to aesthetic injections, and using steroids topically to hide the problem. Although topicals may help, keep in mind that the skin is a protective barrier to keep things out. So any emollients applied to the skin should be USDA Organic Certified. The better and toxin-free the skincare products are, the greater chances to behold a more youthful skin you'll love.

The secret again is to look inside for skin issues. We need to look at what we are feeding ourselves and how that is manifesting itself into good health opening up our gut to infections and microbes that eventually begin to affect the brain, skin, emotions, as well as a whole host of other health issues. Your skin nutrition plan must include the best anti-inflammatory diet and adequate nutrition that supports great looking skin from an inside out approach! We need to simply find the most compatible foods that uniquely support your gut for great looking skin. If your gut is not healthy, you will continue to suffer until the deepest root cause is addressed. So, let's take a look at how to get started.

A few words about hydration. Everyone is pretty much aware that we need to drink ½ our weight in ounces. A good gauge is at least 80-100 ounces of good clean water on a daily basis. Recognize that if the water you are consuming is tap water, it has gone through an average of six other peoples' toilets before it comes back to your home. There is a proverb that states that you can never clean dirty water. Tap water may contain up to 1000 parts per million of total contaminants, which puts a greater burden for your body's innate ability to detox. The best advice is to drink distilled water and supplement with a bioavailable trace mineral. Purchasing distilled water in a plastic container is not recommended, but to invest in a low cost home distiller would be ideal. Search for these on Amazon.

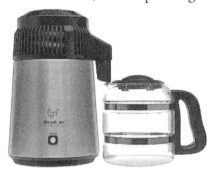

3. Discover Food Sensitivities with DIY Home Testing

I'm sure you've heard of the saying that, "let food be thy medicine, and let medicine be thy food." However, it's also been said that, "one man's treasure is another man's trash." So although broccoli may be good for some, it may not sit well with others. You might be fine with eating nightshades (for example: tomatoes, eggplants, peppers, potatoes, okra, Goji berries), but may cause others skin problems or arthritis. Some people can consume cow's milk (homogenized and pasteurized), but others may be lactose intolerant. Some react to gluten, some do not. One size does not fit all. Everyone's internal terrain is unique to you, your microbiome, and your genetic make up. The point is that you may be experiencing the effects from certain food sensitivities, intolerances, or allergies. Therefore, you may want to consider being tested for food sensitivities/intolerances or just begin by eliminating the most offending foods such as dairy, gluten, lectins, nightshades, and high histamine foods. So once you determine which culprit foods to filter, you may have discovered your sweet spot diet that puts you on a fast-track to better looking skin. Fix your foods, fix your belly, fix your skin!

As mentioned before, not all good foods may cooperate with your microbiome (gut bacteria). The microbiome may be out of balance. When diversity in the gut is lost or out of control, the whole microbial community is affected which creates a cascade of events that manifests itself in other areas of the body like the major organs and the skin. To weed out the offending intolerable foods, a quick at home Food Sensitivity Test can easily be performed using a pulse oximeter or another way to measure your pulse rate. This puts you on the beginning path of determining what foods do not agree with you. Of course, you may have to go deeper, through a functional medicine approach, to actually address an underlying issue if foods are not the culprit, especially if you have tried a myriad of diets to combat bad looking skin.

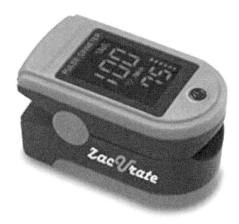

When using a Pulse Oximeter, you will want to record your resting heart rate first. A normal resting heart rate is between 60-82 ppm. When you test a certain food by chewing and rolling it around your mouth for approximately thirty seconds. Then check your heart rate with the pulse oximeter. If that particular food stresses you, your pulse will either go up or down by four beats from your resting heart rate. This would suggest that you may be sensitive to that food and the greater the variation from your resting heart rate, the more toxic the food is to you. Test different foods each day. Any and all offending foods should be eliminated from your diet for at least 60-90 days before re-introducing the food. Now that you've nailed down any foods that may be causing skin distress, and you have eliminated those foods, what's next?

4. Do you have normal labs, but you still feel horrible or still have problematic skin?

You're not alone! So this is what's next…..Grab your labs, even if they are one to three-years-old and let's find out what your blood work is telling us. The answers may be lurking right on the labs that your doctor said were normal. The numbers don't lie! We are simply looking for the CBC with Differential for starters. The

Differential includes the breakdown of the White Blood Cell (WBC) counts. We are looking for the percentages, not the absolute values.
- Neutrophils%
- Lymphocytes%
- Monocytes%
- Eosinophils%
- Basophils%

The functional range we are looking for are the following:
- Neutrophils = 60% Neutrophils fight bacteria
- Lymphocytes = 30% Lymphocytes fight viruses
- Monocytes = 7% Monocytes fight viruses (> 12% suspect Epstein Barr Virus (mono))
- Eosinophils = 3% Eosinophils identify if parasites are a problem, also food sensitivities
- Basophils = 1% Basophils identify also if parasites are a problem

If your lab's values are greater than what is stated, the following are some potential hidden low grade infections that may have been lurking around chronically affecting you for possibly months to even years.
- Neutrophils > 60% (Low grade bacterial infection)
- Lymphocytes > 30% (Low grade viral infection)
- Monocytes > 7% (Viral infection)
- Eosinophils > 3% (Parasitic infection or food sensitivity)
- Basophils > 1% (Parasitic infection)

Therefore, if you are suffering from chronic problematic skin issues, as an example it could be from parasites if your Eosinophil % is greater than 3% or if your Basophil % is greater than 1%. Once you begin to uncover what is hidden in your CBC with Differential, now you can specifically address the underlying issue(s) with all natural protocols, and feel better within ninety days or less. As with all things, resolution may take longer if there are co-infections and other issues that need to be handled, like hormonal imbalances.

What I find most of my patients are struggling with is how to solve their chronic health issues and want to get started on improving their overall health now. They struggle with a chronic health condition for which their primary physician or health care provider has not been able to bring health maladies to resolution, without having to resort to medications. So they get left hanging or jump from one provider to another. At one point in time with my skin issues, I saw eighteen different doctors, providers, acupuncturists, reflexologists, and traveled across the country to see holistic practitioners with no avail to resolving my chronic skin issues. It was finally resorting to a functional medicine approach that made the difference. If you've been like me, this is an area that we focus on, utilizing a functional medicine and functional blood work approach, to get at the deepest root cause of problematic skin. If you are wanting to invest in your health, my contact information is listed below. Improving the quality of your life starts today! My promise to you is that you will get your life back. You no longer need to be a prisoner in your own body.

It's Your Body, It's Your Health, It's Your Choice!

Best Regards and Virtual Hugs!

Dr. Jim

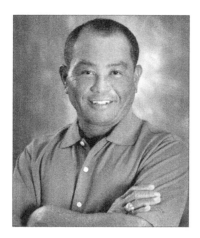

PS–Take the time to ask yourself, did I laugh today? Laughter has been proven to strengthen the immune system. You should have a gut-wrenching laugh every day and smile as much as possible. *A smile is a free gift you can give to someone each day. The smile in return makes you feel good!*

Contact Information:
drhickswellness.com
jameshicks75@gmail.com
james@drjames.coach

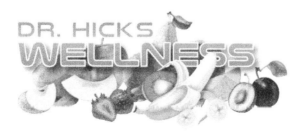

CHAPTER 16:

The Code of YOU

By: Deniece Krebs, CHC

It was Christmas Eve night. Sarah stood in the arms of her husband, paralyzed in fear and hopelessness. That night, in the middle of her kitchen, Sarah was confident that she would not live to enjoy the next Christmas.

I met Sarah a few years earlier at a sales conference and several days after that Christmas Eve night, the LORD prompted me to call her and when she answered the phone, I asked what's going on that I was prompted to call? Needless to say, through tears, Sarah began to tell me about that hopeless Christmas Eve night just days earlier and within twenty-four hours we began working together.

My detective hat went on and together we began to uncover her unique puzzle pieces—the same puzzle pieces that I have used time after time with other "Sarahs" and the same puzzle pieces that I'm going to teach you here.

In this chapter, you too will become your own best health advocate and detective as I introduce each puzzle piece and then at the end, give you a link to my in-depth "Detective Guide" that you can download for FREE—you may want to go ahead and download it now, before you continue reading and then use it as a "workbook" as you read. My objective is to help you discover and understand your unique instruction manual through knowing your DNA and then learn how your lifestyle choices impact those instructions.

When I work with folks, my goals are to:

1. Educate—
    a. Knowledge is only power if and when it is APPLIED. I often refer to this as my "so what" factor. So what...that I know this. So what...does it matter? So what...do I do with this information. So what...does this information impact my life!
    b. Introduce you to the Puzzle Pieces (which I have outlined below.)
    c. Educate deeper into EACH puzzle piece.
2. Expose—
    a. Based on what is discovered through your unique puzzle pieces, we can then identify and expose your blocks.
    b. What does "optimal health" look like to YOU? Not everyone's definition is the same as I discovered with Sarah years after we worked together.
3. Encourage—
    a. You to be your own best health advocate—YOU know you better than anyone (and that includes your doctors!)
    b. You to learn to "listen to" your body, mind, and spirit. This is a discipline, and one worth mastering.
    c. You along your journey—we all hit plateaus and potholes along our journey, but as John Maxwell's books states...we want to fail forward. Learn from every choice's result...good or bad.

4. Engage—
   a. THEN after your education and exposition has taken place, you can then use the seven keys of the Designer's Wellness Plan to unlock your optimal health and abundant life— the fancy word for this is EPIgenetics— the lifestyle choices that impact your instruction manual (DNA) and how your instruction manual's instructions interact with your environment. This chapter doesn't allow us to delve into these seven keys, but I did at the least want to introduce them to you. The seven keys are:
   i. DNA
      1. Know it
      2. Understand it
3. Use it
   ii. Toxins
      1. Reduce Exposure
      2. Remove Existence
      3. Repair Evidence (damage)
   iii. Nutrition
      1. Healthy eating in general
      2. Healthy shopping overall
      3. Healthiest eating for YOU—based on your DNA and goals
   iv. Fasting
      1. Intermittent Fasting
      2. 24-hour fasting
      3. Fasting "schedule" for optimal living

v. Sleep
   1. Power Down Hour
   2. Good Sleep hygiene
   3. Amazing "Sleep Juice" (supplement)
vi. Stress & thoughts
   1. Thoughts do matter
   2. Stress—internal vs external
   3. Breathing to flip the ANS (Autonomic Nervous System) switch
   4. BrainTap® (an amazing tool)
vii. Movement
   1. Why movement is important
   2. Choose the one that you enjoy so you'll be consistent
   3. A little goes a long way

Now that we've covered my four goals for you and listed the seven keys of the Designers Wellness Plan, let's get back to Sarah as I introduce you to each of the seven puzzle pieces necessary for our Detective investigation to be effective.

1. DNA test
2. Detective Guide:
   a. Detailed history
   b. ACE Assessment
   c. Lifestyle Assessment
   d. GUT health assessment
   e. EMF Evaluation
   f. Toxic Burden Assessment
   g. NeuroToxic Assessment

3. Blood lab results
4. Current Toxin exposure(s)
5. Two-week Food/Mood/Poop Journal
6. Optimal Health Spectrum
7. Your personalized plan

As we begin to go through the importance of each of these pieces, let me set the stage and shed a bit of light into my detective brain by sharing these foundational pillars for my life and business:

First of all, Sarah needed to understand the foundational concept that everything impacts everything else. Nothing functions in a vacuum. Everything means everything … every cell, every organ, every system, every choice, every thought. Everything! Remember my "so what" factor.

Next, Sarah had to wrap her head around one simple fact that she is a whole person with interworking and interdependent systems. Although Sarah had a long list of diseases, she is not a disease, a diagnosis, or a label! She was definitely unhealthy, but that is not her identity.

Next, I explained that Sarah was created by a Master Designer and HE created her for a very specific purpose. He has a plan for Sarah's optimal health and abundant life.

Finally, I told Sarah, "*You are a masterpiece because you are a piece of the Master.*"

—Dr. Les Brown

Sarah was now armed with my four foundational pieces and so we could begin exploring each specific puzzle piece.

PUZZLE PIECE 1 - DNA

You may hear health practitioners say they work at the "root cause" and while I initially also adopted that concept early in my health coaching days, I really was driven to the "root of the root" and as I kept asking the question, but why? I finally made it to the true root and beginning. DNA! This is why I call myself the DNA Detective.

DNA, genetics, genome—all basically mean the same although t*echnically* not exactly—this puzzle piece is the unique genetic code that makes you - YOU! We are all familiar with "baby-making 101." Dad's sperm fertilizes Mom's egg. In that sperm is a copy of one of the two DNA code strands from dad and in the egg is a copy of one of the two DNA code strands from Mom. Those two DNA strands come together to create YOU! So, understanding that there are many potential pairings between Mom & Dad provides multiple options and the understanding of how we are each uniquely designed and created.

In order to begin understanding DNA, there are some important fundamental points that I want to cover:

1. Our DNA never changes. Once you get your DNA tested—the results will always be the same (unless future technology comes into play to alter DNA, but we'll leave that for another book)!

2. Our DNA strand contains approximately 23,000(ish) genes and each of those genes is made up of a combination of four proteins totaling enough data to fill 100 encyclopedia *volumes* (that's a LOT of information!) Most of us have all 23,000(ish) of those genes so when you hear language like "I have the MTHFR gene"—you can confidently say "so do I!" (more on that below.) Occasionally, an individual may indeed be born with an extra or missing gene or chromosome, but those situations are very rare.

3. Each one of those genes contains hundreds or even thousands of individual pieces of information that make up that gene. The technical term for these pieces of information is a "nucleotide." Instead of genetic "mutation," the most common type of genetic differences among people is actually a **variant**, not a **mutation/mistake** which is a "single nucleotide polymorphisms," frequently called SNP (pronounced "snip.") The best way to understand this SNP is like a "typo" in the instruction manual.

4. Notice the word *variant* and not *mistake*. I do not like to call it a "mistake" because I do not believe that GOD makes "mistakes"—EVER! These variants are on the single address of a gene (again, a SNP) which can impact the effectiveness of those instructions and on the flipside, our lifestyle choices can impact the effectiveness of those instructions. As noted above, let me give you the rest of the story on "I have the MTHFR gene." The more accurate statement should be "I have a ***variant or variants* on** my MTHFR gene." A variant on this gene can affect the body's ability to process amino acids—namely, homocysteine and that then impacts how the body breaks down and uses B12 and Folate which leads me to this final note about the DNA puzzle piece...

5. SO WHAT! Again, one of my foundational pillars as mentioned above. No matter what you learn or expose in your Detective Journey, let's start to always ask "so what?!" So, what will learning or exposing ***this*** ***information*** do for my action, choice, or impact? If nothing...let's not waste our time! There are so many options that DO have an impact, there is no need to waste time on those that don't.

Congratulations! You are now armed with key foundational tools to discover your first puzzle piece by getting your DNA tested. The next thing to decide is why am I getting my DNA tested? There are basically two camps:

The first camp is what I call the "disease" camp. This is testing for genes that are generally done by the medical community to determine if someone has a truly genetic disease like muscular dystrophy, cystic fibrosis, sickle cell, Huntington's disease, or phenylketonuria to name a few. Over the years, I have found less than fifty truly genetic disease genes in the research and science. THIS is not the kind of DNA testing that is our #1 puzzle piece!

The second camp is what I call the "wellness" camp. THIS DNA testing *is* our #1 puzzle piece. Through this type of DNA testing, we can discover volumes of valuable information toward your optimal health.

It's important that I also share this minor tweak with you—there are some genes that have been made out to be "disease" genes that I categorize as "wellness" genes. One of my favorites to share is one that Sarah immediately commented on when she said, "I think that I have the Alzheimer's gene." I love exposing this one, because the gene being referred to, "APOE" (Apolipoprotein E) and is actually a gene on nutrition panels as it has to do with instructions for how the body processes saturated fat. If your manual's instructions aren't effective and efficient for how your body processes saturated fat, then you have an increased likelihood of a potential buildup of saturated fat which could then lead to cognitive problems. So, you see, APOE is not a gene *of* a cognitive decline disease, but the *result* of lifestyle choices around what that gene is designed to do based on your Designers Wellness Plan! Let me go a step farther. If Sarah discovered that she had one or two variants on her APOE gene, then we would simply adjust her saturated fat intake and incorporate activities to help the body process the saturated fat so we decrease potential build up! Viola! *That* is the "so-what" factor in action.

As with Sarah, we learned that she was much more susceptible to toxins because her body's inflammatory response was not the greatest; her vitamin D receptors would naturally function well in absorbing vitamin D from the sunshine and effectively transporting it to her cells; her immune system needed support; her body's free radical defense was not optimal; her detox pathways didn't function optimally; her body's preference for protein, carbohydrates, and fats; how her body processed of a host of micronutrients like Vitamin A, B, C, E, K, Selenium, magnesium; and so much more! THIS is the type of rich information we want to discover about you as well because armed with *this* kind of information allows us to answer the "so what" factor when we get to puzzle piece seven and create your plan.

Now that we know the *kind* of DNA test that we want allows us to decide *which company* to use for testing. As of the time of print, there are likely at least one hundred companies offering to test your DNA. Be informed when deciding which company to choose. I personally am not a fan of 23AndMe as in recent years they have changed the genes for which they test and we don't gain as much knowledge on our wellness "so-what" information as what I prefer to learn.

Here are seven questions to ask when choosing a DNA testing company:

1. Do they use certified equipment and methods fit for the task?
2. Is the DNA testing lab CLIA certified and CAP accredited? This ensures accuracy and privacy of your results.
3. Is your genetic and personal information handled and stored safely?

4. What will the company do with your DNA? Will they sell it? Use it for research?—if any of these, we might want to run away.
5. Who owns your genetic data and results? You or the company?
6. Are the results based on reliable scientific data that is kept current?
7. Do they give you clear results and reports that can be used for action steps?

As with Sarah, we knew why we were testing her DNA and because I had already evaluated the companies, we got her DNA tested, received back her results, and incorporated those results when we put her plan together!

Congratulations! We now have our first puzzle piece collected and are armed with an arsenal of very helpful and useful "so-what" information unique to YOU.

PUZZLE PIECE 2 – Detailed History

While we waited for Sarah's DNA test results to come back, which usually takes between two and four weeks, we moved on to the next puzzle piece through utilizing a very comprehensive "***Detective's Guide***" which is FREE to you (the link will be at the end of the chapter so you can download and begin your own detective journey—be aware…it is <u>very</u> comprehensive and may take about an hour to fully complete)!

Sarah completed the Detective's Guide which covered topics such as her detailed history (not just health history, but life history,) GUT health, EMF Evaluation, ACE (Adverse Childhood Experiences) assessment, toxin exposure, and a lifestyle review. As mentioned earlier, we are a whole person with cells, organs, and systems that all work interdependently with one another so when you see questions about root canals, silver fillings, birth control usage, or camping—know that there is a reason, and each question is another important "a-ha" for me when connecting your dots!

Let's remember foundational pillar number one...everything affects everything else! Unless we can turn over every piece of the puzzle, we cannot get an accurate picture of YOU!

With such a comprehensive assessment, it allows me to do my favorite part of my "detective work" which is to connect dots. I still remember the zoom call with Sarah when I showed her life's timeline and was able to back track her history of symptoms and feelings of unhealthy to a job she had thirty years earlier when she was exposed to fumes in an unventilated copy room all day, every day. This exposure created a toxin overload in her body because her DNA instructions weren't effective in removing those toxins; therefore, each following internal and external stressor that happened for the next thirty years simply over-taxed her body's ability to detox naturally and thus began the compounding health challenges and the ever-growing list of diagnoses she collected from a long list of health professionals.

That moment was Sarah's "a-ha" moment and my clarity to know where to begin with her seven keys to the Designer's Wellness plan.

PUZZLE PIECE 3 – Recent Blood Lab Results

While Sarah's first two puzzle pieces gave us a significant part of her picture to optimal wellness, we did have a few more pieces to add.

Next is blood work.

For years, clients would send me their bloodwork results and want me to shed light on those results for them and for years, I gladly accepted them as I knew there *were* clues, but wasn't exactly sure how to find them nor what they were. I even enrolled in a certification course to learn it all. While that course was fantastic, the chemistry was WAY over my head and as hard as I tried to keep my head above the intellectual water, all I did was frustrate myself. One of the most impactful pieces of information that I did learn from this course, ironically was in the very first class and is something that not only surprised me, but honestly, angered me. That is —when the "big boy" labs print off your results and you look to the right side of the line, you'll see a column titled "normal range."

If you learn nothing else in this chapter, please allow what I'm about to tell you next to be burned into your memory and tell everyone you know!

"Normal" does not mean "optimal" nor "functional" — "normal" does not equal "healthy!"

You see, in that first blood chemistry course years ago, I learned that "normal," when it comes to labs' reporting, more closely means AVERAGE! These are really "reference" ranges, a bell curve of 95% of the population and then deemed "normal." The upper 2.5% and lower 2.5% represent abnormal blood test results. Apparently, labs add all tests of a particular marker done over the past given time frame (say one year or five years) and AVERAGE the results to create this "normal range!" If these "normal" ranges are based on 95% of the population…do I want to be "normal?"

When I explained these following two examples to Sarah, she had another "a-ha" moment!

White Blood Count (WBC) on the Complete Blood Count (CBC) panel:

"big boys" labs say "normal" is that this number should be between 3.4 & 10.8 however, optimal and functional tell us we want this number between 5 & 8.

Sarah's number was 4.3 which meant that all of her traditional health practitioners said—"All good! Sarah, your labs are **normal**!"

This left Sarah frustrated and hopeless, yet again. However, from my "optimal" detective lens, I said… "Hmmm…Sarah, it looks like your body may be fighting some type of "foreign invader" of a low-grade infection. Let's dig a little deeper to see if we can find out if that "foreign invader" is in the virus/bacteria/fungus world or parasite world or "man-made" chemical or toxic metal world so that we have a targeted plan of attack. In Sarah's case—parasites were her "foreign invader" along with chemicals and toxic metals.

My second favorite example of the comparison between "normal" and "optimal" is Vitamin D.

"big boys" labs say "normal" is between 30 & 100; however, optimal and functional tell us that this number needs to be above 60 because the body needs the hormone D for over 400 processes in the body and 30 just won't cut it—if you don't have enough, the processes aren't able to do their job and some functions will lose beginning the cascade of health challenges.

Sarah's Vitamin D? Twenty. In this case, by both "normal" and "optimal" ranges—she was below the number, but sadly, the majority of traditional health practitioners don't even look at Vitamin D unless you, the patient, request—and in some cases—DEMAND to test it.

Once I learned this incredibly valuable piece of information along with what IS the "optimal" or "functional" range—NOW, this puzzle piece has much more significance in our Detective journey for both Sarah and all my other "Sarah's."

Although that one piece of information was priceless, I still didn't feel comfortable or confident including bloodwork with my client's Detective journey; however, I was in practitioner group with Dr. Kylie who would occasionally host a workshop that I'd jump on and slowly began to understand more about the clues found in bloodwork!

Now, I can confidently look at bloodwork results and expose presence of low-grade infection and determine if that infection is from viruses, bacteria, or parasites by reviewing their CBC. We can expose evidence of leaky gut and how well your detox system is working by reviewing your kidney, liver, and adrenal numbers in your CMP, know if your body needs Vitamin D and so much more.

This puzzle piece also works in partnership with your DNA test to show if your body is expressing a genetic variant or another clue on the type of vitamin or mineral supplement that your body does best with (normal or converted "methylated" form.)

With Sarah's blood work, we could add the puzzle piece that confirmed her DNA was weak in inflammation and immune function which provided another confirmation to the root cause culprit of her un-health again pointing to her job decades ago when she was exposed to some toxins that her body simply could not process and therefore likely led to her leaky gut which continued the cascading effects that now had her hopeless in her health crisis standing in her kitchen that Christmas Eve crying in the arms of her husband.

PUZZLE PIECE 4 – Toxin Exposure and Burden

This puzzle piece may very well be my second most favorite one, although, if I am honest…I love them all because they are all important to success, optimal health, and abundant life! Know that this is a **HUGE** puzzle piece and contains potentially hundreds of smaller puzzle pieces which means that it is an ongoing piece to explore and expose. Unlike previous puzzle pieces that are a one-time discovery, this is one of lifetime exploration and constant pivoting.

As we begin to explore and expose this puzzle piece of toxins, allow me to introduce you to a strategy that I developed years ago called the **SOS** strategy.

SOS - Swap Over Stop.

When Sarah and I began to explore toxins that she was being exposed to, she, like all of my other clients immediately said... "***don't make me give up* _____*!*** [fill in the blank for yourself.]" Sarah's "blank" was wine. She and her husband loved exploring wine country and creating memories with wine tastings. My response to Sarah was the same as with every other client. I will not ***make you*** give up anything!... but would you consider my SOS strategy?

Are you open to swapping your wine for a better, non-toxic choice? Sarah responded as I expected...of course! This SOS strategy has led me to explore many products and categories so that I can confidently and effectively provide great swap suggestions regardless of the product such as make-up, foods, wine, coffee, healthy lifestyle tools, water filters, sleep aids, and more. Did you know that coffee and wine are the two most toxic beverages that we can consume!? Fear not – I have a better choice for you.

So, with that commitment, Sarah and I walked through my "detox your life" strategy which systematically goes through five areas of life where we are exposed to toxins, sadly more often today, we are **UNKNOWINGLY** exposed.

Let's look at these five areas together: kitchen, bathroom, home, soul, and environment. Because each area has so many smaller pieces, for the sake of time and space, I have selected two of the most impactful suggestions or tasks as a best or better choice in each area to help kickstart your own detective journey to optimal health.

Before we dive into each area to detox, we must first lay the groundwork of "**Toxins 101**." I needed Sarah to understand what defined a toxin? She immediately went to the common definition of a toxin which was something like fallout from a nuclear bomb. "No way! I've never been around any toxins!" Then, I shed some additional light—a toxin is anything your body doesn't recognize or can't use. This could even be something that is generally <u>good</u>, but <u>bad</u> for you! I like to split toxins into three main categories: living organisms, non-living things, and good stuff but bad for you.

"Living organisms" would be things like viruses, bacteria, parasites, fungus. They are alive, but either should not be in your body at all or should be in your body, but have gotten out of control or gone rogue. Bacteria is a great example. We have more bacterial DNA in our body than human DNA and that's actually GREAT! Those "good gut bugs," as I call them, have a very special job in our body which is to breakdown and absorb nutrients, but when they grow out of control or the bad gut bugs take over the good gut bugs, bacteria is now toxic. Sarah understood that and turned out she had some of the bad living organisms in her body in the form of parasites that she had contracted years ago.

The next category that Sarah and I discussed was "non-living things" which is a rather large category and covers man-made things like chemicals and plastics plus natural elements like metals that are natural, but shouldn't necessarily be in our body. Lead, for example, is a good metal, but when it's in our body causes some major issues especially with our thinking. This was one of Sarah's toxins. As for chemicals, I can't think of one that is helpful circulating in our body but sadly are quickly becoming an epidemic for many. These would be pesticides, herbicides, and pharmaceuticals. While pharmaceuticals are used for addressing issues in our body like uncontrolled blood pressure or blood clots, they are all chemical, synthetic, and patented copies of ingredients that God made. Please don't hear me as an anti-drug flag-waving person! I am not. It's just that I prefer pharmaceuticals as the last resort and choose to focus on supporting the body to do what God designed it to do in the first place. With Sarah and all other clients, we do not deal with pharmaceuticals, but all the other "non-living" toxins that are present yet should not be. If we could identify with Sarah what was causing internal stress at her cellular level and remove it (or them) then she would be able to better handle the external stressors of life.

Lastly, the category of "good stuff but bad for you." The most common place this category shows up is with food. Dairy and wheat are **good** but due to the current condition of your body may be **bad for you**. The great news in this for Sarah was that her long list of "good, but bad for you" pertaining to foods eventually dramatically reduced and she was able to enjoy them again with no issue.

Now that Sarah was armed with Toxins 101 and could easily identify a toxin, we could then move into a handful of foundational principles so that she could implement my SOS strategy. Here are the general *principles* that I taught Sarah to determine "Is It Toxic?"

1. "If/Then." If God made it, then it is likely non-toxic. If man made it, then it is more likely to be toxic. Please keep in mind that this is a principle, not a rule. There are items on both sides of these If/Then principles that are contrary to the principle, but generally speaking, we can use this as a starting place in evaluating, "IS IT TOXIC."

2. The next principle has to do with the ingredient list on the back of the container. The fewer ingredients the better so when choosing packaged products, choose the ones that have less ingredients, preferably without some form of sugar at the start of the ingredient list. Sarah had a love for licorice. She searched and searched to find the best licorice available, both in taste and ingredients, eventually finding a brand that had only four ingredients and those ingredients were whole organic foods—this would be like "grandma made" if your grandma was a licorice maker.

3. The compounding effect. While research and government agencies may deem a single chemical ingredient "safe," we

must keep in mind that the more ingredients we add together through multiple products the higher we increase the compounding effect. Think of high school chemistry class. Eventually, there was one ingredient that caused the otherwise calm liquid to bubble, overflow, or explode. Each element of that chemistry experiment was by itself "safe," but combined became toxic, explosive, and potentially deadly. Have you ever combined vinegar and baking soda? If you have not, do not create this concoction as a drink, but it is a great drain cleaner! We see this principle play out most often in make-up and bathroom products layering several products together creating the compounding toxic effect.

4. And the final principle as introduced above - SOS Strategy. Swap Over Stop. If there is something you just cannot live without such as coffee, wine, or ice cream, swapping it for the best choice is a win!

Sarah was now armed with the definition of a toxin along with these simple principles, so we began to detox her five areas starting with her Kitchen Detox.

Detox Your Kitchen—Our kitchen has so many places to detox, but let's look at the two on the top of my list. Food and plastic.

First regarding foods. Get familiar with the Environmental Work Group's (EWG) annual list of the ***Clean 15 and Dirty Dozen*** [link: https://www.ewg.org/foodnews/full-list.php]. This tool makes it incredibly easy to choose the best selection of whole foods based on how they are grown. While the best choice is organic whole foods and local regenerative farmers so that you get to know the farmer and their farming practices to be sure they do not use pesticides or herbicides; however, budgets don't always allow for this "best" option. So, the better choice is to utilize this resource from the EWG to choose organically/regeneratively grown items listed on the "Dirty Dozen" and feel comfortable choosing items on the Clean 15 that have been "conventionally farmed." This is a great way to help live healthy on a budget and begin to remove toxins from your kitchen. At the bare minimum, the "good" choice is to move to more whole foods and away from packaged and processed foods which will reduce toxic exposures immediately as a result of processing.

Sarah learned this and began to search for local farmer's markets and pay attention to whole food selections at local groceries so that she and her husband could take this first step toward reducing toxin exposure through what they ate.

Second kitchen area to detox is this easy rule (*Yes! I said "rule!"*) **Never put plastic and food together when heat is involved.** Period.

I gave Sarah a few examples of what this looked like, and she quickly got it. Placing leftovers that are still hot/warm in plastic containers. Drinking water from plastic water bottles that have likely been in a truck or on a dock in the heat of the day or left in your car. Hot coffee in plastic cups. Restaurant's to-go orders or leftovers in plastic or styrofoam containers. And the one that Sarah almost missed…when cooking, don't use plastic utensils to stir hot sauces or flip things in the skillet.

If Sarah understood the "why" then the detox was easier to implement. When heat meets plastic, the heat changes the molecular structure of the plastic and can allow exchange of the food and plastic. Plastic is known as a "xenoestrogen"—it looks like the hormone estrogen to our cell's estrogen receptors and when our cell's estrogen receptors are locked with fake estrogen (plastic,) then the real estrogen can't get in and be used resulting in hormone crazies and problems! If you have ever put spaghetti sauce in a plastic container, you have witnessed this first-hand. The plastic container is forever stained with the red of spaghetti sauce. Wonder what also went into your spaghetti sauce?! Yep! Plastic molecules. Implement the rule of **Never put plastic and food together when heat is involved.**

Detox Your Bathroom—The bathroom is likely the area where we are exposed to the most toxins so again, we have a long list of items to evaluate and implement the SOS strategy, but to get Sarah started quickly, we focused on two things. Antiperspirant/Deodorant and make-up.

First—antiperspirant/deodorant. When Sarah and I first began working toward her optimal life, there were very few good Aluminum-free deodorants available, but today, we have more choices. We still need to scrutinize the ingredients on the back label and not just trust the front marketing so get in the habit of reading the ingredient list and aluminum-free (or all metals for that matter) is a must. Our pits are full of pores which are very close to many lymph nodes. Lymph nodes are part of our lymphatic system whose primary job is garbage collectors and eliminators throughout our body. The last thing we want to do for our lymph nodes is to cake on toxic metal and then seal those pores (antiperspirant) to trap in our garbage.

When Sarah was ready to swap antiperspirant for an aluminum-free deodorant, I suggested she do it over a long weekend when she could actually "detox her pits." If you are like Sarah, during this "Pit Detox," things will get a bit stinky! To help with this process, Sarah used a green tea and charcoal face mask on her pits to draw out the toxins faster and added a few activities to help flush her lymphatic system since it does not have a pump of its own like the circulatory system has the heart to pump.

Those activities included rebounding (jumping on a small trampoline or simply the act of bouncing up and down on your tippy toes as if you were on a trampoline), dry brushing (using a slightly stiff dry brush to lightly brush your skin starting at your ankles and working your way up your body always brushing toward your heart), and tongue-scraping (using a copper tool that is shaped like a "U" to gently scrape off the gunk from your tongue each morning before eating or brushing your teeth and rinsing the gunk down the sink). These activities helped her lymphatic system to start moving better as it had become sluggish from decades of antiperspirant use and toxin exposure. Sweating is also a good thing! It is part of the body's natural detoxing process so to block that process keeps toxins in our body. This is why dry infrared saunas are so wonderful—they force the lymphatic detoxing system to rid the body of toxin build-up.

The second area of the bathroom, especially for women, is our make-up. Every time we put make up on our faces, we are introducing hundreds of chemicals and toxins into our bloodstream within twenty-six seconds. That is how long it takes for anything we put on our skin to enter our bloodstream. While there are not as many non-toxic makeup choices as there are deodorants, there are a few. The Environmental Work Group is another great source for discovering these products. The EWG has a pretty fantastic app for both foods and skincare.

Detox Your Home—While both the Kitchen and Bathroom are in the home, this category covers the entire home. As with the kitchen and bathroom, there are many many areas we can tackle, but here, my top two for greatest impact. Cleaning and water.

First, cleaning products. Once Sarah understood ingredients and toxins from our Kitchen and Bathroom Detox, it didn't take her long to immediately recognize the number of toxins she was cleaning with and immediately implemented the SOS strategy. My favorite choice is to make my own DIY cleaning products using essential oils and safe household ingredients like vinegar and baking soda; however, there is also a fantastic company that I love called Norwex who provides some incredible toxin-free cleaning products that I suggested to Sarah. I often have a catalog show going with my gal, Michelle White.

The second area for the greatest impact in our Home Detox is water. While you may be thinking, "water? Shouldn't that belong in the "Kitchen Detox?" Yes, it is, but water is everywhere. We drink it. We cook with it. We clean with it. We shower in it. As we discussed with food selection, we will again look at good, better, best.

Where water is concerned, in my opinion, the bare minimum is the "good" in our ***good–better–best*** scale which pertains to the water Sarah drank. The minimum requirement in every home who wants to move to healthy, optimal, and abundant living is to filter the water you drink and with which you cook. Sarah immediately bought a countertop water filter and only drank water that came out of that filter. There are good electric ones as well as good gravity-fed choices. You'll need to determine which one is right for you and your family, but no matter which one you choose, be sure to confirm that it is filtering out ***all*** the bad guys: metals, pharmaceuticals, fluoride, chemicals, and sediment. Including a reverse osmosis filter in your water filter selection is also a good option so read the details of the water filters that you research.

The "better" choice in our ***good-better-best*** scale is to also filter the water coming out of your shower head and faucets in addition to all the water with which you drink and cook. In Sarah's case, her most toxic exposure was from her nightly hot bath soaks in her toxic water when she was sitting in her 200-year-old bathtub that had a crack in the porcelain and lead from her houses' old lead water pipes and lead paint dust which was all leaching into her body night after night after night when her pores were opened from the hot bath. When Sarah made just this one change, she immediately began to feel much better since we were taking her through a total body detox at the cellular level, she was not constantly exposing her body to more toxins faster than we could remove those stored in her body.

Best option would of course be a whole house water filter that will remove the hundreds of chemicals, pharmaceuticals, and toxins found in nearly every city water source across the country from ALL water in your home. That choice is a pricey one but certainly the best.

Detox Your Soul—This next area can be a bit of a challenge as it is often not visible and it is personal which is always harder to see in ourselves. While Sarah was doing a fantastic job in all other areas, this one was going to be her most challenging as it tends to be with most. As usual, there are many specific things, but the two with the greatest impact are going to be other people and our thoughts.

Detoxing your soul is so challenging because many times, toxic people are close to us—that is why they are toxic. If they weren't close to us, their own toxic lives would not spill over and become toxic to us. Because toxic people tend to be close to us, we must learn how to create a bubble so that their toxic life choices just bounce off us. Believe me, I know this is MUCH harder to tackle because it requires a constant conscious choice, and we must be vigilant to know how to allow toxic people into our life (if we must) without allowing their toxic lives to penetrate our emotional life. If possible, stop spending time with those people; if that's not possible, then it requires emotional boundaries and intentional conversational choices with them. You get to determine the topic of conversations when with them and can take the lead in conversations or you may need to be more direct by protecting your mental health and saying, "I love spending time with you, but I would respectfully request that we talk about things that are encouraging and move us to being better, healthier, and happier."

This brings us to the second part of Detoxing Your Soul—your own thoughts. The key to Sarah's success in tackling her own toxic thoughts was to implement our SOS Strategy again because Sarah had adopted stinkin' thinkin' about herself which is not uncommon when a person feels so terrible for so long and sees no hope in sight. So, Sarah and I went back to the basics. We had to dig into the truth about who she is and adopt that while repelling all other comments or thoughts—whether from herself or others.

Rewiring the brain DOES work!

Detox Your Environment—Environment can mean many things and yes, it's logical to think about our work environment that may be damp or moldy—surrounded by toxic fumes in a factory which are definitely part of our environment and necessary to evaluate when we are detoxing our life. But I'm going to focus on something that we can't see, but our cells definitely feel!

Digital devices' and the toxins in our airwaves. More importantly, the proximity of your digital devices to your body. Specifically, your phone. Please please please, keep your phone at least one foot away from your body when at all possible. While I generally don't like to give "don'ts" as action steps, in this case, it might be easier. This topic of electronics and WiFi has been somewhat controversial and requires an entire workshop which we don't have time for in this chapter, so for now, please take my word and just implement these two rules (yep! said rules again!) and one guideline:

- **Rule #1:** Do not keep your phone in your pants pocket, bra, or waist band...don't carry it "on" your person. On rare occasions, it's ok, but not on an ongoing regular basis. Consider this logic, your phone is always sending and receiving information via WiFi. If those signals are going out near your breast tissue, sexual organs, or gut, those parts of your body are in the path between your phone and the signal "out there," so they are being blasted. The blasting does absolutely affect your cells.

- **Rule #2:** Do not sleep with your phone under your pillow or on your nightstand close to your head. Charge it at night in a different room! Again, the signal is blasting through your brain if it's under your pillow and at the cellular level, those signals are keeping your cells active and alert so that they are unable to do what your Designer intended to be done at night—rest, digest, repair, heal, and catalog.
- **Guideline:** If your home's WiFi router is near anyone's bedroom—turn it off at night. Your body needs to be able to rest and constant WiFi signals don't foster rest, repair, and healing. If you cannot turn it off, can you move it or shield it from the bedroom?

Want to guess where Sarah's home's WiFi router was? At first, her response was common, "OK, we're good—it's downstairs!" But, when I asked one more question, we had another light-bulb moment. "Where is that downstairs room in relation to your bedroom?" The silence told me we had another puzzle piece come into clarity. So, beginning that night, Sarah and her husband turned it off each night and sleep improved; therefore, rest, detoxing, and healing also improved.

That gives you a small glimpse into this massive puzzle piece. Remember, unlike our other puzzle pieces that are a quick test or assessment, the puzzle piece of toxin exposure is an ongoing one for which we must constantly be aware of making ongoing small course corrections. Again, I've put together entire courses around Detoxing Your Life! That is the importance of detoxing.

PUZZLE PIECE 5—Two-week Food/Mood/Poop Journal

This puzzle piece is often the most difficult one to expose. It isn't that Sarah was unwilling to do it and it's not hard. She would often simply forget as most of us do with this piece; however, this one is so important because sometimes certain foods don't cause a problem immediately as we once suspected. I ate this and then had digestive problems within thirty minutes to one hour. Bingo. Problem solved. Food sensitivities *used to be* an immediate "if/then" situation; but not so much anymore. Food sensitivities can take three to five days to cause problems and by then, we've forgotten what we ate three to five days ago which is why keeping a two (or four)-week journal is key to exposing how certain foods affect our mood and poop. It just might not be what you thought!

It is not a difficult process, only challenging to remember to log every single thing that goes into your mouth. Sarah was no different, she would walk past the counter, break room, or refrigerator and without thinking, grab something and pop it in her mouth. It wasn't until we began to see a pattern that showed up about two and a half days after she would eat an actually healthy food that she would tank—she would get such brain fog that she could hardly drive. While that food was a good "healthy" food, it wasn't good for HER! Once she eliminated that food, her brain fog also began to lift and she celebrated another milestone win on her optimal health journey.

While we are on this Food/Mood/**Poop** Journal, allow me to take a moment to stress the importance of pooping. Ideal pooping should be daily, preferably two to three times each day, but definitely not two to three times per WEEK and absolutely not every other week! It is very important that your body voids waste, otherwise we create an entirely new kind of toxin in our body—our own biowaste. Have you ever driven by a dead animal on the side of the road—out here in the country we have lots of deer that get hit and boy do they stink. Imagine the same meat and other foods rotting in our bodies because we aren't pooping it out.

One other thing that I want to mention while we're tracking the poop part of your journal is to pay attention to your poop. I realize it may sound gross, but all moms of babies do this every time a diaper is changed. I still remember my sister being a bit of a detective over twenty years ago as she changed her boys' diapers to see how she needed to tweak their next few meals…more grapes or more bananas she would tell me. Little did I know what an impact those comments would have on my life as I would then become the DNA Detective!

That's it for this puzzle piece. It is a short one, but a very important one indeed. There are many ways to do this. Good ole fashioned paper and pen, an electronic note on your phone, or there are a few good apps out there, choose the one that fits your schedule and personality the best. This Food/Mood/Poop Journal puzzle piece is more about getting it done than how it's done.

PUZZLE PIECE 6—Optimal Health Spectrum

Let's quickly recap Sarah's journey. It's now been three weeks and we have her DNA results in hand, she's completed her comprehensive Detective Guide, received back blood work, began identifying toxins and utilizing the SOS strategy, finished her two-week Food/Mood/Poop Journal so we are now ready for perhaps her key puzzle piece. This is the one that will guide not only her plan, but Sarah's drive. This one is the piece that I missed with my clients for many years until my business coach, Dr. Russ Rosen, introduced it and changed my entire practice. Dr. Russ is one of the most impactful Business Coaches with whom I have ever worked! [http://theohcsystem.com/]

Before the two questions, first, the foundation – your definition. Dr. Russ gave us a scale of negative ten (at death's door) to zero (I'm "OK." Nothing really "wrong" or I'm not on any prescriptions, I'm just "OK") to positive ten (off the charts living my best life, feeling amazing, conquering the world.)

Please keep this important tidbit in mind. <u>My definition</u> of "negative 3" or "positive 5" or "zero" may look different than <u>your definition</u> of "negative 3" or "positive 5" or "zero." Like a pain scale that you may be asked by a medical professional, "On a scale of 1-10, what's your pain today?"—your definition of a 3 on your pain scale may be what I would call a zero or +10 on my scale. It does not matter the number to anyone but you— this is YOUR Optimal Health Scale! If you know what a specific number looks and feels like to you, then you will also know what the improvement of that number looks and feels like to you when we get to the second question below.

Dr. Russ gave us a helpful chart below with descriptions of various categories of health as a "guide" not the definitive rule.

OK, now we are ready for the two questions.

First—*where are you today* on this Optimal Health Spectrum? Are you a 0? +3? -8? You determine the number based on how you define the scale's numbers. Write it down in the margin or put an X on the scale below.

```
|-----------------------|-----------------------|
-10                     0                     +10
```

	ENERGY	STRESS	SLEEP	PHYSICAL	MENTAL/ EMOTIONAL
OPTIMAL +8 to +10	Vibrant Energetic	Extremely Adaptable	Optimal Sleep	Peak Physical Health	Joy, Happiness Zest for Life!
EXCELLENT +4 to +8	High Energy	Handle Stress well	Excellent Sleep	Feel good Strong, Flexible	Positive & Happy Clear thinking Good memory
GOOD +2 to +4	Up & Down Energy	Up & Down Stress	Good Sleep	Occasional Feel good most of time	Feel good, slight fog & memory trouble
COMFORT ZONE +2 to 0 to -2	OK Energy	Average Stress	Moderate Sleep	Feel OK Occasional minor pain	Emotional Ups & downs Brain fog & memory trouble
FAIR -2 to -4	Tired	Moderate Stress	Fair Sleep	Constant aches pains & symptoms	Slight depression Anxiety, Irritable
POOR -4 to -6	Fatigued	Extremely Stess	Poor Sleep	Chronic disease Occasional acute episodes	Moderate depression or anxiety
AWFUL -8 to -10	Exhausted	Cannot Cope	Severe Insomnia	Serious Chronic disease/illness frequent acut episodes	Serous depression or anxiety

Perfect! Question two. Using this same scale, descriptions in the chart above, and YOUR definition…*where do you want to be?* REALLY! Don't just pick +10 because you think you should. What does "optimal health" mean to you and your life? What is <u>*your*</u> goal for "optimal health?" (Not my goal for you or your significant other's or parent's or children's…) **YOUR goal for YOUR optimal health**. Give it a number on the same -10 to 0 to +10 scale.

Excellent, note that number in the margin to the side or put a smiley face on the same scale above.

As mentioned earlier, this was the piece of Sarah's puzzle that I missed. Sarah was making tremendous progress and had begun working again. You see, she was in such bad shape when we began working together that she couldn't even work anymore. She was feeling better, her relationship with her husband was beginning to thrive again, her symptoms were fading away into a bad memory. Then, all of the sudden, Sarah stopped working with me and I was shocked, hurt, very confused, and of course took it personally that I had "done something" that caused her to not want to work with me any longer. It wasn't until about three years later when I began working with Dr. Russ and he taught me this very important puzzle piece that I had *my* own "ah ha" moment. What would Sarah have said if she had the opportunity back when we started working together?

You guessed it—I called Sarah and after catching up on life, I asked her…Sarah, I know it's been a while since that Christmas Eve night years ago and you're not the same person as you were then, but I'm wondering, if you were to think back to that time and you had a way to determine where you were on this scale between -10, zero, and +10 (and I gave her some descriptors in the chart above,) where would you have scored yourself?

"Deniece," she said. "I thought I was going to die! Negative TWENTY."

WOW Sarah! Thank you so much for sharing that…so where did you <u>want</u> to get? "I just didn't want to die," was her response. "I would have been thrilled with **negative two!**" I was a bit confused as my expectation was that she (and everyone) wanted to be at +10. Since she said a negative two, GOD told me to ask one more question which has become the most important question for my understanding and work with my clients.

OK then. Sarah, where do you think we ended up? Her response floored me, and I learned a tremendous amount from mine and Sarah's conversation. "I was at a positive two or three." [insert mic drop]

That was the day and the conversation that I decided to add this very important puzzle piece to my detective toolbox. You see, the reason Sarah stopped working with me was that she had far surpassed her internal and possibly subconscious goal of a "**negative two**" and was now living in the "**positive** two-three" so she didn't need me anymore, but I just didn't know that because I had not incorporated this puzzle piece when I was working with her. SHE knew she was feeling better than she dreamed possible, even if it may have been at the subconscious level.

Now, how about you? Where would you put yourself today and where do you want to be? The beauty of this puzzle piece and every other one is it is personalized to you. No answer is wrong. Your definition of "optimal health" and abundant living is your definition. Not mine. Only you know what your life's purpose is and what it looks like to live that purpose and what your life feels like today in your own "unhealth." Regardless of your goal, I will do everything in my power to help you achieve it.

On a side note, Sarah is not alone in reaching a number on that scale that is beyond her hopes and dreams. I remember another client (whose goal was +5) and after our first ninety days working together, we checked in on her Optimal Health Scale when she hit that "5" and I said, "fantastic! So, we're done?" "Heck no!" she quickly exclaimed, "I'm not stopping now. I've had days when I felt like +20…I'm going for +10 every day! I didn't think it was even a possibility, but now that I see it is, I want that to be my normal."

The Sarah's of the world are why I love being the DNA Detective with my clients to guide them in educating, exploring, exposing, and engaging their personalized optimal health and abundant life.

PUZZLE PIECE 7—The Plan

In some cases, we need to add a few other puzzle pieces which generally looks like additional testing of gut health, a few more blood lab markers, or some deeper toxins, but for the most part—that's it. We now have all pieces of your puzzle as well as the picture on the box top—where you want to be on that Optimal Health Scale from -10 to +10. Now it's time to put your plan together. While everyone's plan has similar building blocks, the exact look and feel of your building blocks and the potential order of building may be slightly different.

For example—everyone is dealing with various form(s) of what I call "foreign invaders," but the kind of foreign invaders are different. Do we need to address viruses? Bacteria? Parasites? Toxic metals? Tick-borne critters? Mold? Chemicals? Or likely a combination of these as many destroy in partnership with one another and one toxin makes another foreign invader opportunistic.

Everyone's plan includes these seven keys: DNA, Detoxing, Nutrition, Fasting, Sleep, Stress & Thoughts, and Movement. When we dive into each of these keys, we don't try to tackle them all at once and we begin with the one that makes the greatest impact fastest. Sometimes these keys require supplementation and sometimes they offer opportunities for better choices but most of the time, they involve both.

Sarah wholeheartedly adopted one of my favorite quotes by Maya Angelo, "***Do the best you can until you know better. Then when you know better, do better.***" Sarah became her own best health advocate, not accepting answers from her medical professional who said, "that's just how it's going to be," or "there's nothing that can be done." When Sarah explored her puzzle pieces with me, she became a force to be reckoned with! Not even her husband could get in her way. Renewed hope and vision drove action. Several times she would call me with a new way to discover a toxin, finding environmental testing kits to evaluate water, lead, air, etc. to determine exactly what was poisoning her. Her journey possibility even produced a new passion. Sarah got a taste of abundant living and wanted more as she began to dream again of those dreams for her life of days gone by because now hope has a new home.

This chapter isn't long enough to outline each of the keys for the plan, but I've dropped tons of videos into a DIY online vault. However, before you start watching those videos, if you are like Sarah and want to become your own DNA Detective to begin exposing your own puzzle pieces, I invite you to visit www.TheCodeOfYOU.com/your-guide and download this free guide and get started today.

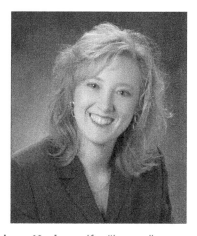

Hello, I am **Deniece Krebs,** wife, "bonus" mom, daughter, sister, sister-in-law, favorite daughter-in-law, aunt, great-aunt, friend, and most importantly, daughter of the Most High King JESUS. I love working with women to help them discover and live their purpose while journeying along them on their personalized optimal health path to a giddy gut, happy hormones, and hope restored so that they can relive their honeymoon every day. Over the years, I have added to my toolbox certifications in health coaching, essential oils, epigenetic human performance, detox specialist, and functional blood chemistry specialist. At the end of the day, I am your DNA Detective with my company called The Code Of YOU and love using my "crazy brain" (as my dear friend Cindy called it one day) to help you discover your puzzle pieces and connect your dots to create your optimal health and abundant life as part of the Designers Wellness Plan! Thank you for reading and owning your own best health!

CHAPTER 17:

Depression & Anxiety and the Thyroid Connection

By: Jessica Watterud, LPCC

Depression and anxiety have almost become common in our society. Most of us have either battled ourselves or know someone who is currently struggling. According to the National Institute of Mental Health (NIMH), 21 million adults and 4.1 million adolescents had at least one episode of Major Depression in 2020 with the rate being higher in females. NIMH also estimates 31.1% of adults will experience an anxiety disorder at some time in their lives. Females are also at higher risk for an anxiety disorder. (NIMH, 2020)

Anxiety is a normal human emotion. Everybody experiences anxiety. Without it, we would never get anything done. We would not correct behavior. Anxiety prevents us from getting too comfortable and remaining stuck. For example, if we do not feel anxiety as a due date approaches on a project, we are less likely to get it done. We do not like the feeling, so we do something to remove or reduce it. The problem is anxiety can get out of control. When anxiety rises to the level of Clinical Anxiety, it is now interfering with our ability to function in our daily life.

Clinical depression also interferes with a person's ability to complete tasks of daily living. People throw that word around a lot, and it can lose its meaning. Clinical depression is more than sadness. Depression is consuming and takes over the mind and body. Depression is painful, both physically and mentally. People do not just "get over" depression. Depression, like any other illness, needs attention and care for the individual to get better. It takes time. It takes consistency. It takes work. Often, what is helpful in treating depression is the opposite of what the person wants or has energy to do.

When an individual gets a diagnosis of depression or anxiety, they may get medication. Hopefully, they are involved in mental health counseling. An effective counselor will help a person get to and heal the root of the symptoms. What often is missing when a person is struggling with symptoms of anxiety and/or depression is the search for the underlying issue. It is easy for us as providers to look at the symptoms related to our own field and either ignore or refer to another provider for the symptoms that seem unrelated. But what if they are all related to one another?

Let me tell you a story about a young man who was twenty-three-years-old at the time I worked with him. We will call him Steve (name has been changed). He did not remember a time in his life when he was not depressed. Steve did not recognize it as depression as a child but looking back he said all the signs were there. He reported he spent most of his adolescence in the basement of his house playing video games. He did not do well in school because he did not have any motivation to do his work. His major complaints were trouble sleeping and low mood. As you can imagine, Steve struggled in multiple areas of his life. Holding down a job was difficult because he struggled to get out of bed. He did not have relationships outside of his family and even those were strained. With such a long history and the severity of his symptoms,

Steve was looking at long term therapy and potentially medication. Steve did not want to take medication again. He had tried several and, in his opinion, the side effects were worse than depression.

Typically, in a case like this, I would begin with getting a good sleep routine, some coping tools for stress and improving mood, and improving relationships. All of these are helpful tools for improving anyone's mental health. The most frequent complaint of someone coming into my office is difficulty sleeping. Figuring out what is going on with sleep can be like a chicken or egg conversation. Which came first? Is anxiety/depression creating poor sleep? Or is poor sleep creating an anxious and/or depressed mood? Either way, working on improving sleep will naturally improve mental health. Our bodies and brains need sleep for all the systems to work properly. Without sleep, we struggle to concentrate, it is harder to manage emotions, our immune system is less effective, and the list goes on and on.

Let us go back to what Steve did. Steve began supporting his body through supplements, nutritional changes, and exercise. Within a few months, there was a noticeable difference in him. He was smiling, making new friendships, got an excellent job, and was moving out on his own! All the things we would have spent months working on in therapy began to happen naturally. His sleep improved. He was able to handle daily stressors. He had energy! It changed his life.

I am a huge believer in mental health counseling, obviously. And when we treat issues in isolation without thinking about how everything is connected, we miss important clues. Steve and I could have spent twelve months or more working on ways to improve his life. And I do believe he would have benefited. We did spend those few months finding tools to help him manage stress and take care of his mental health. With both together, Steve was able to heal faster and get his life back.

Our bodies are incredibly interconnected. You cannot treat the mind without treating the body. One of the first things I talk with my clients about is taking care of their physical body so they can do the work to heal their mind. What I have noticed repeatedly is that when clients are physically healthier, they naturally begin to heal mentally. This does not mean there is still no work to do. But the clients who are taking care of their bodies are more likely to engage in the work needed to heal mentally. Almost all of them, when they notice a slip back into old mental patterns, will identify that they need to get back to taking care of their body because that was when they felt the best. Additionally, the clients who are not taking care of their bodies take much longer to do the emotional work needed to heal and some are not able to get there. Think about how you feel when you have a bad cold or stomach flu. Can you recognize what is going on with your emotions and take care of them? Probably not. You are more likely to just take care of your physical needs because that is the highest need right now. Your body will prioritize the same way. If your energy is needed to fight a low-grade bacterial infection or virus, your body will focus there rather than on other body systems such as calming your nervous system so you can sleep.

Ideally, when a person seeks treatment, the provider would be requesting some minimal bloodwork to rule out physical issues when there are symptoms of anxiety and/or depression (something we call "best practice"). There is a strong connection between thyroid issues and mental health issues. If you were to do an online search for the symptoms of hypothyroidism, depression is listed as one of them. Also, many of the symptoms of hypothyroidism are the same as the symptoms of depression. However, if you were to search for hyperthyroidism symptoms, one of the symptoms is anxiety or nervousness and many of the other symptoms would overlap with the criteria required to get a diagnosis of an anxiety disorder from a mental health provider. This is a huge factor to consider when treating mental illness. Look at the overlap of mental health diagnoses and an imbalanced thyroid:

Anxiety/Hyperthyroidism	**Depression/Hypothyroidism**
Weight loss	Fatigue
Increased heart rate	Weight gain
Nervousness/anxiety	Muscle weakness
Appetite changes	Muscle aches, tenderness, stiffness
Fatigue	Depressed mood
Shaking	Memory problems
Sweating	Slowed heart rate
Muscle weakness	
Sleep problems	

There is a strong connection between chronic stress and disease. This is not a new concept but with our western medical model we have gotten away from looking at all aspects of a person's life. What tends to happen today is primary care doctors will refer to a mental health provider after all medical interventions have failed or when all tests come back "normal". People who experience high physical and/or emotional stress in their lives are more likely to develop chronic disease later. Stress weakens the immune system and throws the body systems off balance. Our stress response system was designed to handle temporary stressors. When we are under elevated levels of stress for prolonged periods, the system cannot regulate and get back to calm. We stay on high alert, sometimes without any awareness of it! This elevated state puts the body into chaos. Multiple systems are impacted such as the digestive system (your gut), the circulatory system (your heart and blood vessels), the endocrine system (your thyroid, adrenals, and hormones), etc. As you can imagine, it is equally as important to support the body's system in getting back in balance as it is to reduce stress.

One metaphor I use often is thinking of our life like a plate. We only have so much room on our plate, and we may have a different size plate than someone else. For example, my four-year-old uses a smaller dinner plate than my eleven-year-old who uses a smaller dinner plate than myself. I also put less food on my four-year old's plate than on my eleven-year old's plate because they have different capacities. It is the same for our mental and emotional capacities. We all have the same number of hours in a day, but maybe you can take on more than me without feeling overwhelmed. That is ok. We each have different size plates. Maybe tomorrow you cannot take on as much as you could yesterday. That is ok too. We have different capacities on different days.

This metaphor is used often, and people will talk about removing things from their "plate" to reduce stress. That is something to consider. There may be things we can remove even if it is just for a brief time while we heal. What if there is nothing to remove? What if typical daily stressors are just overwhelming?

Learning how to rest is a key factor in how much stress we can handle both physically and emotionally. Just like I mentioned earlier about sleep, our bodies require rest to function properly. Some cultures do a much better job of this than most western cultures. And guess what? They also have much lower rates of most health-related issues including anxiety and depression.

When I looked at my own "plate" there just was not anything to remove that would make a significant difference in my stress levels. There is also a level of stress that comes with even the good things in life at times. So, if we cannot reduce the stress outside, we look at the stress inside. By finding what is impacting the body and mind from the inside we can reduce overall stress without having to remove outside stress. In the ideal situation, we can remove the internal stressor and reduce outside stress to get the biggest impact.

If you're looking for some things you can do right now to start your healing journey, start here:

1) Change one thing to take better care of your body (drink more water, get some more movement, get outside, etc...).
2) Schedule time for rest. It does not count if you are sitting down working on something. Find something that is truly restful and make it a priority at least once a week.
3) Examine your "plate." What can be removed or reduced?

Now I am going to tell you my own story. I was thirty-four-years-old. I had four boys. I was exhausted. I do not just mean I needed to take a nap sometimes or go to bed early. I mean I could never get enough sleep. I would sleep nine hours and struggle to stay awake on my drive to work. I was functioning on large amounts of caffeine. I had to work extremely hard to focus. My work suffered but worst of all my family suffered. I was so irritated all the time and my children and husband paid the price. I told my doctor that I wanted my thyroid checked. She told me it is normal to be tired. I am a busy mom with young kids. She was partially right; I **was** a busy mom with four kids! But I knew my body, and this was not right. I argued until she did the bloodwork. And everything came back to normal except Vitamin D was low. Most of the world is deficient in Vitamin D so this was not surprising. I started taking Vitamin D and did not notice much of a difference.

Then my wonderful friend told me about someone who read her bloodwork a different way, developed a supplement plan that supported her body, and got her back to healthy. I contacted this provider and went through the process. I could not believe the results! I didn't even know I could feel this way. I woke up feeling rested. I was able to enjoy my kids. I had energy to go outside with them in the middle of the afternoon and work in the garden or push them on the swings. I was able to be the mom I wanted to be. I decided soon after that I needed to learn how to do this. How many other people were struggling just like me and being told their symptoms were either normal or were given pill after pill to take care of the symptoms without taking care of the root cause? I knew I was not alone.

Does any of this sound familiar? Maybe it's you that has been struggling. Maybe it is someone you care about. If you have tried everything and just are not feeling better, it might be time to try something different. I have a five-day challenge for you to get better sleep than you are now. Getting quality sleep is an important part of healing.

www.pathtowardhealing.com

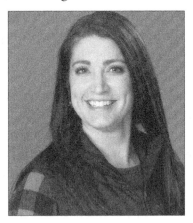

Jessica Watterud is a Licensed Professional Clinical Counselor in the state of North Dakota. She is a Certified EMDR Therapist and Functional Bloodwork Specialist. Jessica has been in the mental health field for the past thirteen years and has been in private practice for seven. She is a mother of four boys and lives on a farm with her family, two dogs, several cats, and chickens. Jessica loves spending time on the farm, camping, reading, and running to all her boy's activities.

CHAPTER 18:

Your Health Puzzle

By: Renee Swasey

Navigating pieces to put the puzzle together

Do you feel health is scattered puzzle pieces, always searching for conventional and non-conventional healthcare professionals, therapies, and remedies to help you connect the pieces to maintain or regain your health? Overwhelmed listening to the "gurus of health" on what to be eating, drinking concoctions, taking test after test with no tangible answers, or all of this with hopes to be the solution to the whole puzzle, as frustration sets in as pieces aren't fitting or questioning if they are part of your puzzle at all?

Yep, I can relate. Knowing bathroom locations was my priority every time my foot stepped out my front door. Tiredness and fatigue was my level of energy. Financial debt set in trying things to get healthy. Family time or events were missed or limited because of mental war thoughts I had in putting myself in situations that heightened anxieties. I was uniquely masquerading living a healthy lifestyle because my profession was helping people with their health.

It was 2007 when I heard a sermon titled "Running on Empty" that resonated with me and started the change from the inside out.

A life that I thought looked like I was in total control, but I was running on empty, grasping strains on the end of my life rope and chaos raging within me. That's where my true healing began, and I hope my chaos, my mess, and my test will encourage you to heal beyond the diagnosis.

I have been in the natural health field since 1994, with head knowledge, but was not practicing what I preached to clients. I wasn't applying protocols I had learned on myself. This will sound crazy, but I thought, hilariously, since I have the knowledge that's all I need to be healthy, but that's not how it goes.

For me it took, and continues to take faith, patience, self-control, applying knowledge, and doing the work. Health is a constant journey and is never a destination. I desire to have more life in my years because we aren't guaranteed more years to our life.

In 2017, I was introduced to food inflammation testing to offer clients, as my symptoms above exacerbated and was affecting my home and career life, this was the first test and service I actually followed through with personally and was one of the many pieces to my health journey. I would worry about needing to excuse myself during sessions with clients to use the restroom, and anxiety heightened just thinking about it at the beginning of each session. After one week of knowing the foods that I needed to stay away from, I saw a huge improvement, which I knew was a piece of my health puzzle.

I continue to test every year to tweak what is needed, even though my bathroom anxieties were resolved.

In 2019, I felt like a tin woman in need of an oil can to lubricate every joint, muscle, tendon, and ligament. Every day my legs were as tight as tree trunks. I had severe discomfort, including cold hands and feet, along with a bundle of other symptoms. I was getting massages every week, every other week chiropractic sessions and avoided foods from my inflammation testing. All of these were helpful but I felt like something deeper was going on inside my body.

If only I could get a full body scan of some kind, I thought. That's when I remembered a test I had undergone years prior called Thermography, that I hadn't paid much attention to results. Remember I never followed through and in the past did not apply what I knew.

Thermography is a physiological test, which demonstrates thermal patterns in skin temperature. Results may either be normal or indicate disease or another abnormality. Thermography provides you with an image you can see in real-time and can indicate areas that are afflicted or have improved. This knowledge enabled me to know what was working for me and what changes needed to be made with my personal health goals and treatments.

On March 10, 2019, I had a full body thermography session and I learned that I had peripheral vascular insufficiency. In other words, poor blood flow.

A registered nurse encouraged me to learn about micro-circulation, a type of therapy that enhances blood flow and encourages the body to heal itself. The sessions are done fully clothed while lying or sitting on a mat that enhances microcirculation. Movement of the blood at the capillary level brings oxygen and nutrients to the cells and tissues. At the same time, toxins and wastes (like carbon dioxide) are removed. I thought, why not give it a few months? This sounds like what I need.

On April 20, 2019, I started to use the device at home before introducing it to my clients. After two months and a lot of research, I felt I had increased energy. The cold feeling in my feet and hands seemed to decrease, along with the numbness in my fingers. I no longer felt like a tin woman in need of an oil can. From July to August

2019, I started to feel phenomenal, with increased endurance, more energy, and less discomfort. I began to be more active, especially with my family. I started riding a bike and hiking with them, which I had never done prior. I felt so phenomenal that on Aug 22, 2019, I had to see if my result would show up visually. They did! Another piece to add to my health puzzle! (Check out my before and recent pictures at Alleghenymuscle.massagetherapy.com).

Our bodies are always changing and adjusting because of internal and external stressors. The need to continually re-evaluate what pieces work or don't work in our health is part of putting the puzzle together. For example, food inflammation testing and microcirculation are two pieces of my health puzzle that work for me.

You may be asking yourself, "where do I start?" Here are six pieces I call the *Pillars of Health*. I will briefly go over them to help you navigate and evaluate where to start in your health right now and what to focus on to take the first steps. They do not go in any certain order because of the nature of the different stages of life we each live. Natural health is simple and mundane rather than a quick fix. It is slight habits that lead to success—so you may ask," why doesn't everyone not do them?"

It's easy to do but just as easy not to do, you pick your easy, or in other words, it's hard to be healthy but just as hard to be sick .... pick your hard.

FIRST PILLAR OF HEALTH—Mind and Emotional /Spiritual Growth

Your mind is powerful. Thoughts you think, words you speak and emotions you either try to hide or fully express are part of natural health.

What are your thoughts about your health right now? How about the words out of your mouth? Are they full of hope or despair? Are you still holding on to the past that may be affecting your health now? What is the battle going on in your mind that may be a barrier to your breakthrough?

Here are a couple of examples: as a licensed massage therapist, people would come in with a pain in their neck and in conversation, they may express that something or someone was a "pain in their neck." Another example is when people say, "I've tried everything." I have to ask, "why are they here with me?" Are they just going to try it, or actually be ready to follow through with the full experience that would bring them to a breakthrough of change and healing?

My personal story: I suffered from gluttony. I ate when I was happy, sad, angry, or mad. I thought about food constantly, from what was going to be offered at an event or celebration, to that piece of cake or cookies I would reward myself after an accomplishment of some sort. Food was my idol.

Listen to what you're saying and thinking, and that may be just where you need to start to piece your health puzzle together.

Remember, natural health is simple and mundane. Doing something to improve your health little by little each day which, in time, will lead to results and success.

Here are a few tips if you feel that this is the pillar you need to start with:
- Monitor what's going into your mind—ask yourself if this is going to renew your mind or have no value.
- Fast from or decrease watching the news or TV shows—replace that with reading ten pages of something that will renew your thinking, encourage you to grow into a better mindset.
- Distance or limit yourself from emotional drainers- we all have them in our life. Also be aware if YOU are one!
- Journal the thoughts you think, the words you speak and emotions you feel. Also what barriers are stopping you from having more life in your years?

SECOND PILLAR OF HEALTH—Nutrition

Remember natural health is simple, mundane, and consistency is key—it's easy to do and just as easy not to do, it's not a quick fix.

We all eat and need food so the question is, do you live to eat, or are you eating to live? What are you filling your grocery cart up with? Living foods or dead foods? Are you listening to the media and gurus, or listening and getting to know your body by how it feels and reacts when you consume food? Are you just plain outright confused? To keep it simple, at least 80% of our food choices daily should consist of living foods, which are: If it falls from a tree, grows from the ground, runs in a field, swims in the water, or flies in the sky, if the food can reproduce on earth, then it will reproduce in you.

If it has an "ingredient label," it should consist of nutritional-dense foods and not chemicals, preservatives, or additives. You may think, "I'm so busy, eating healthy is not quick and convenient." Think about it, you're running out the door, is it quicker to grab an apple from the fruit bowl on the table or open a bag of chips? Just about every grocery and convenience store has pre-cut veggies, fruits, and single servings containers of avocado, hummus, and more healthy options other than foods that are not real and that are C.R.A.P. (C=Carbonated Drinks, R=Refined Sugars, A=Artificial Foods, P=Processed Foods).

It's just as easy to open a bag of veggies as it is a candy bar wrapper. Are you listening to what you are saying to yourself in silence or out loud to those around you when you say, "oh I shouldn't be eating this?" If so, listen to yourself and don't eat or drink it. If eating healthy is still a struggle in your thoughts, revisit pillar one and journal what the barrier might be in renewing your thinking.

Again, it's easy to do, but it's just as easy not to do.

THIRD PILLAR OF HEALTH—Hydration

When our garden, plants, or grass needs hydration, we don't go and reach for the soda can, alcohol bottle, juice bottle, or milk container, we get the hose or water can to feed them. Hydration is so important for many functions such as detoxification, temperature regulation, keeping mucous membranes moist and transport of nutrients. How much should you consume a day? Half of your body weight in ounces is suggested per day. Divide that by hours in a day and set a timer every hour to drink a calculated amount to reach half of your body weight in ounces.

FOURTH PILLAR OF HEALTH—Sleep/ Rest/ Stress Relief

Sleep is when the body detoxifies, repairs, and recovers. When our body gets enough sleep we have better mental alertness, energy and overall well being.

Helpful tips and resources:
- Limit bright lights, including electronic screens such as TV, cellphone, and computer after sunset. Avoid at least thirty minutes prior to bed.
- Practice diaphragmatic breathing.
- Don't eat a heavy meal late in the day, but also don't go to bed hungry.
- Tart cherry is a natural source of melatonin which can bring on the feeling of sleepiness.
- Lavender essential oil on a pillow, towel or diffuser can help calm the body.
- Read a book (not on a screen!) before bed. Remember to choose reading material that will renew you!

FIFTH PILLAR OF HEALTH—Movement

We simply need to move. Movement helps internal organs, muscles, joints and overall health. Start somewhere. There are free resources everywhere online to get moving and active. If the only thing you can do is walk ten steps, then start there! Be honest with yourself, if traveling to a fitness facility is time consuming then start with an activity at home.

SIXTH PILLAR OF HEALTH—Elimination (physically and mentally)

We are bombarded with toxins every day, both physically and mentally. It's important to eliminate these toxins from our bodies. Keeping our liver, bowels, urinary tract, lungs, and skin functioning will help keep our body running well. Keeping the mind clear from toxic thoughts is just as important (see pillar one).

Gut health is essential as viral, bacterial, fungal infections and parasites can wreak havoc on our system. Symptoms are not the problem, they are a result of an underlying problem, and addressing gut health may alleviate symptoms that you may be experiencing.

In conclusion, all pillars work together, depending on where you are in your life, one or two pillars may need to be addressed to balance out the others. You need to start somewhere and if finances are an issue, start with one suggestion given in that pillar that resonates with you the most. If finances are accessible, my suggestion is to test rather than guess. Testing such as blood labs, thermography, food inflammation testing, and other tests can help you understand what state your body is in and what it needs to regain health. This book may be a great place to start in finding a practitioner that you resonate with!

Still don't know where to start putting your health pieces together? I'll leave you with this story: a father was reading the morning newspaper while his little daughter played on the floor next to him. There was one problem, the father wanted to finish the article he had started but the little girls' cheerful interruptions prevented any reading. Glancing around, he spotted a possible solution. A magazine was lying beside him with a map of the world. "Here, honey," he said to his daughter. "Daddy made a puzzle for you to put together and see if you can make a map." With that, the father returned to his article, confident he'd have plenty of time to finish the piece he had been reading. In no time at all, his daughter said, "Daddy, I'm done!" Surprised, he looked down to find the map fully assembled. "That was fast," he said. "How did you put it together so quickly? You don't know anything about geography." His daughter replied, "there's a picture of Jesus on the other side of the map. I knew when I had Jesus in the right place, the whole world would be all right!"

For me and my personal journey, I had to start with pillar one, that sermon in 2007, "Running on Empty" was a piece of not only my health puzzle but my life puzzle. What pillar do you need to start with in your health puzzle? Remember, it's easy to do but just as easy not to do. Pick your easy or in other words, it's hard to be healthy but just as hard to be sick...pick your hard. Health is a constant journey and choosing to have more life to your years is your choice. Praying your health chaos turns into change, your health mess becomes a message of hope, and your "testing," both physically and mentally, becomes a testimony of a life transformed so you can start healing beyond the diagnosis.

You can find me at Alleghenymuscle.massagetherapy.com

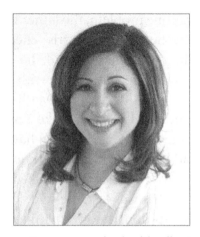

Since 1994, **Renee Swasey** worked with clients ranging in age from newborn to elderly with massage and since 2003 with Naturopathy. She has worked with hospitals, hotels, spas, chiropractors, student and professional athletes, professional companies, and individuals like you who are working toward achieving their health related goals. Her training encompasses Board Certified Naturopathic Practitioner, Functional Blood Lab Specialist and licensed Medical Massage. She has taught massage at both the college and trade school levels and has lectured publicly on health and quality of life benefits achieved through natural health, muscle therapy and massage. She has been married since 1997 to her husband, Scott. They have a son and daughter. Her life verse is Proverbs 3:5-6 because when she does things her way, it never works out but when leaving it all to God, a miracle unfolds each day and gives Him the glory and not herself.

CHAPTER 19:

Microscopic Maestros

By: Mike Rhees

The Astonishing Ways Your Microbiome Conducts the Symphony of Your Body

John, 52, was grappling with uncontrolled Type 2 diabetes despite medications and regular monitoring, leaving him perpetually fatigued. Upon discovering an article about the microbiome's role in diabetes management, he delved into the relationship between gut health and insulin sensitivity. Eager to take action, John consulted a functional medicine doctor to incorporate gut health strategies into his diabetes regimen.

Under his functional medicine doctor's guidance, John made dietary changes and used specific therapies aimed at nurturing a healthy gut microbiome. Following this regimen diligently for several months yielded astonishing results: his energy surged, blood sugar stabilized, and A1C levels dropped. John's life took a positive turn as he felt rejuvenated and regained control over his diabetes.

John's remarkable turnaround is just one example among many, as the microbiome's role in chronic and autoimmune diseases is extensive. Comprising not only bacteria but also fungi, viruses, and other microbes, the microbiome is a vibrant ecosystem that acts like a perfectly tuned orchestra, with each microbe playing its part in maintaining the body's systems.

This microbial symphony plays a vital role in protecting against long-term and autoimmune diseases, and also positively impacts different parts of the body with its varied microbial members. The sheer size and diversity of the microbiome, and its substantial effect on our health, are highly significant. Maintaining a balanced microbiome is important not just for bacteria, but also for the fungal and viral components of the microbial community.

The growing area of microbiome research is uncovering its crucial role in chronic and autoimmune illnesses. While many mistakenly think it's mainly about solving digestive problems like constipation or Irritable Bowel Syndrome, the microbiome's wider influence on the whole body is often clouded by misunderstandings and not fully recognized.

Jamie, a 38-year-old graphic designer, faced challenges in work and personal life due to chronic fatigue. Seeking solutions, she consulted a clinical nutritionist and herbalist who attributed her fatigue to an imbalanced gut microbiome. A holistic plan was devised, which included dietary changes to eliminate refined sugars and processed foods, a detoxifying protocol for her GI tract, and therapies for restoring her microbiome diversity and intestinal health. Within weeks, Jamie saw improvements in her energy levels, and after six months, she experienced a remarkable reduction in fatigue, rekindling her ability to excel at work and cherish her family time.

To tap into the microbiome's power in fighting autoimmune and long-term diseases, it's important to grasp the concept of dysbiosis. Dysbiosis throws off the balance in the microbiome, leading to a decrease in good bacteria and a proliferation of harmful bacteria. Dysbiosis can also involve an imbalance of fungal and viral populations within the microbiome. This imbalance can negatively impact digestion, weaken the immune defenses, and create problems in various body systems, highlighting the importance of a balanced microbiome for overall health.

When there's an excessive growth of harmful bacteria and other microorganisms in the gut, they generate toxins and cause chronic inflammation. This weakens and damages the intestinal mucosal barrier, commonly known as the gut lining. This damage impairs the lining's ability to effectively allow nutrients to be absorbed while preventing harmful substances from entering the bloodstream, a phenomenon often termed "leaky gut".

Leaky gut triggers an overactive immune response, which can lead to the onset of Irritable Bowel Syndrome (IBS), Crohn's disease, celiac disease, chronic fatigue syndrome, fibromyalgia, arthritis, and even mental health disorders such as depression and anxiety. Managing dysbiosis and therefore managing the integrity of the gut lining is crucial in preventing and addressing these conditions.

Dysbiosis can weaken the immune system's ability to fight infections and may even contribute to the development of allergies and autoimmune diseases. A weakened immune system due to dysbiosis can make the lungs more susceptible to infections and may exacerbate conditions like asthma.

Mental health is also greatly impacted by dysbiosis, leading to issues like anxiety, depression, and cognitive decline, often referred to as the gut-brain axis. Dysbiosis can impact insulin sensitivity, leading to metabolic disorders such as Type 2 diabetes, and can also affect the thyroid and adrenal glands. Dysbiosis has also been linked to higher levels of certain substances that can lead to clogged arteries. This makes the cardiovascular system more susceptible to heart disease and stroke.

Dysbiosis can cause inflammation which can manifest on the skin, leading to conditions like eczema, psoriasis, and acne. The balance of microorganisms is also crucial in the urinary tract and reproductive organs. Dysbiosis can lead to urinary tract infections and, in menopausal and postmenopausal women, can negatively impact the changes associated with menopause.

During menopause, there is a significant drop in estrogen levels. Estrogen is known to influence the composition of the microbiota in various parts of the body including the urogenital area. As estrogen levels drop, the composition of the microbiota can change, which may contribute to dysbiosis. A healthy microbiome during **menopause and postmenopause** can help maintain vaginal tissue integrity, reducing the risk of infections, and support nutrient absorption essential for bone health and metabolic regulation. This contributes to a more balanced physiological state, mitigating some of the adverse effects associated with hormonal changes during this period.

A wide-range of chronic and autoimmune conditions are closely tied to an imbalance in the gut's microbiome. Fortunately, restoring balance in this microbial community is achievable. Employing a thoughtful combination of natural therapies, dietary modifications, and a diverse selection of probiotics and prebiotic fibers can foster resilience in the gut and promote the health of various bodily systems, including cardiovascular, hormonal, nervous, skin, brain, and immune systems.

As part of the specific dietary modifications, prebiotics are specific fibers and compounds that stimulate the growth and activity of the beneficial microbes in the gut. Foods that are rich in prebiotics include *garlic, onions, leeks, asparagus, apples, seaweed, chicory root, artichokes, jicama root, avocado, fennel bulb, sweet potato, beetroot, and nectarines*. Prebiotics serve as food for beneficial bacteria in the gut and encourage the growth of various beneficial bacterial species, thereby promoting a more diverse and resilient microbiome.

Probiotics, sometimes called microbiota, bacterial species, or flora, make up a rich and diverse community. There is, in other words, a vast world of probiotics, now found in therapeutic dietary supplement options, that benefits the sheer size and diversity of the microbiome. Incorporating probiotic therapy and diversity into a regular lifestyle is the cornerstone for holistic wellness, ensuring our internal ecosystem flourishes and dynamically adapts to the ebb and flow of life's demands.

When it comes to autoimmune diseases, the makeup of the microbiome is connected to the development of **rheumatoid arthritis**. Having certain bacteria in the gut can trigger inflammation that hits the joints. By restoring a balanced microbiome through diet therapy, specific probiotic species like lactobacillus rhamnosus and salivarius and bifidobacterium bifidum and breve, and other lifestyle interventions, the gut can help regulate the immune system and alleviate symptoms of rheumatoid arthritis.

In the study titled "Expansion of intestinal Prevotella copri correlates with enhanced susceptibility to arthritis" published in Arthritis & Rheumatology, scientists discovered a link between gut bacteria and rheumatoid arthritis. By studying stool samples, they found that people who recently got diagnosed with rheumatoid arthritis had a lot more of a certain bacteria called Prevotella copri compared to healthy people. This study highlights how the gut's bacteria might play a role in rheumatoid arthritis and opens up new possibilities for finding and treating the disease by focusing on gut bacteria.

There is evidence to suggest that alterations in the gut microbiome may play a role in the development of **Type 2 Diabetes.** Promoting a healthy microbiome through targeted remedies can be a complementary approach to managing metabolic health and insulin sensitivity. For individuals with Type 2 Diabetes, modifying the microbiome through dietary changes and targeted probiotic therapies can improve glucose regulation.

One notable clinical study was published in the journal Nature in 2012, under the title "Gut metagenome in European women with normal, impaired and diabetic glucose control." It revealed that the gut microbiome is crucial for insulin sensitivity and glucose metabolism in Type 2 diabetes patients, as their gut flora shows a diminished capacity to digest key carbohydrates. Intriguingly, the study demonstrated that through strategic dietary changes, such as an increased intake of a variety of probiotics and foods rich in prebiotic fibers, there was a marked improvement in insulin sensitivity among the diabetic individuals.

This diversity of fiber consisted of non-starchy vegetables such as *broccoli, brussel sprouts, spinach, carrots, chia seeds, avocados, artichokes, collard greens, and pumpkin*. These specific foods are not only rich in fiber, but specifically in prebiotic fibers. Prebiotic fibers are non-digestible parts of foods that act as food for the good bacteria in the gut.

The gut microbiome's role in modulating the immune system suggests that it may play a part in the development or progression of **Multiple Sclerosis (MS)**. Rest assured, studies have indicated that altering the gut microbiome through diet and supplementation can affect the course of the disease.

The special link between the gut microbiome and Multiple Sclerosis (MS) was emphasized in a 2017 study in the Proceedings of the National Academy of Sciences. The study showed that people with MS have different gut bacteria, especially lower amounts of good bacteria like Prevotella and Sutterella. The results suggest that these differences in bacteria might be linked to the inflammation and nerve-related symptoms seen in MS. The study also pointed out the possibility of using diets high in prebiotic fiber to increase healthy bacteria and lower brain inflammation, opening up new ways to handle MS by focusing on the gut microbiome.

People with **Celiac Disease** can find relief through a balanced microbiome which aids in nutrient digestion and reduces inflammation from gluten.

Emma, 32, was diagnosed with Celiac disease in her late twenties after suffering from chronic fatigue, abdominal pain, bloating, and weight loss. Despite adopting a gluten-free diet, she continued to struggle with symptoms and nutrient deficiencies. Her functional medicine doctor recommended an autoimmune friendly (AIP) diet coupled with a focus on gut health through probiotics and prebiotics. By consuming a nutrient-rich autoimmune diet and cycling through a variety of high-quality probiotic supplements, Emma experienced substantial improvements in her symptoms within a few months, including increased energy, reduced abdominal pain and bloating, and healthy weight gain.

As another debilitating and common chronic illness, **Chronic Fatigue Syndrome (CFS)** is linked to gut microbiome composition. Specific types of probiotics and prebiotics can mitigate chronic fatigue and support adrenal function. Lactobacillus and Bifidobacterium strengthen the gut mucosal barrier, which in turn protects the mitochondria by preventing toxins and inflammatory substances from entering the bloodstream. As these particular probiotic species and prebiotics keep systemic inflammation at bay, energy is improved due to elevated ATP production. Prebiotics are fermented by gut bacteria to produce short chain fatty acids, which in turn impact energy levels via mitochondrial production of ATP.

Bifidobacterium infantis 35624 is a special probiotic that can help CFS patients, especially since they often have irritable bowel problems. Another one, Lactobacillus plantarum, was highlighted in a 2016 study for helping with the mental fatigue part of CFS. These probiotics are a hopeful new option for helping with the symptoms of CFS.

Turning our attention to another vital aspect of our physiology, the "gut-lung axis" explains the symbiotic relationship between the well-being of the gut microbiome and lung health. A 2017 study in the European Respiratory Journal explored the role of the gut microbiome and its connection to immune responses in **asthma**. Researchers observed that changes in the gut bacteria composition were linked to the frequency and severity of asthma attacks. They found that certain bacteria strains produced short-chain fatty acids, which had anti-inflammatory effects and reduced the frequency and severity of asthma attacks. This suggests that a balanced gut microbiome may be a key component in managing asthma and improving lung health.

It's important to note how a healthy microbial balance throughout the body is a surefire way to help with inflammatory conditions pertaining to the **skin**. In fact, specific inflammatory skin conditions are a result of dysbiosis, or bacterial overgrowth of the skin. **Rosacea, psoriasis, dermatitis, eczema, rashes, stretch marks** and other issues pertaining to the skin, are each impacted by a diverse microbiome or lack thereof.

As an autoimmune skin condition, psoriasis has been linked to dysbiosis of the vast skin microbiome. There are specific microbiota species that are the most abundant in healthy skin flora. In addition to specific diet interventions, specific probiotic species such as Lactobacillus rhamnosus, Lactobacillus fermentum, and Lactobacillus salivarius have been studied for their anti-inflammatory properties, which can be beneficial in managing psoriasis.

Rest assured, it's possible to restore the most predominant types of microbiota of the skin and thereby improve the skin's immune properties. For example, bacillus licheniformis produces antimicrobial peptides that protect the skin from infections and also helps the skin to maintain moisture and protect against environmental irritants. Other unique skin specific microbiota/probiotics, called Propionibacterium freudenreichii, bifidobacterium lactis HN019, Lactobacillus rhamnosus HN00, and Lactobacillus sakei all have amazing therapeutic properties. These involve calming down skin irritation and redness and preventing the overgrowth of harmful bacteria, fungi, and viruses. Having antimicrobial properties, they also help defend against pathogens and can be beneficial in the prevention and treatment of skin infections. They also help the skin absorb nutrients and improve skin hydration and elasticity. Involved in the breakdown of sweat, they help in the management of body odor. Last, but not least, they support the skin's defense mechanisms against environmental stressors, including UV radiation.

In a 2014 Nutrition Reviews study, supplementing Lactobacillus salivarius LS01, a predominant bacteria of healthy skin, was shown to alleviate eczema by fortifying the immune system and harmonizing gut flora. Furthermore, a 2023 study highlighted the prowess of another skin probiotic called Lactobacillus reuteri NCIMB 30242 in bolstering skin elasticity and hydration. Collectively, these studies highlight the potential of targeted probiotics for skin wellness and the management of dermatological conditions.

The interdependent relationship between the gut microbiome and the **immune system** is crucial for safeguarding against infections and diseases. Key probiotics boost natural killer cells and generate antibodies that create an environment inhospitable for harmful bacteria. Additionally, the probiotic yeast called Saccharomyces boulardii strengthens the intestinal barrier, blocking toxins and pathogens from entering the bloodstream.

Probiotics like Lactobacillus helveticus and Saccharomyces boulardii engage with the immune cells in the gut, bolstering white blood cells' activity and strengthening the intestinal walls, as shown in studies published in the Journal of Dairy Research and PLOS ONE. These probiotics also expertly modulate inflammation and boost cytokine production, which are essential in immune response. The symbiosis between these beneficial microbes and the body's defenses highlights the vital role of a balanced gut in sustaining a strong immune system.

The **cardiovascular system** also benefits from a healthy microbiome. Certain bacteria help break down dietary fiber into short-chain fatty acids, which have been linked to reduced risk of heart disease. Additionally, the microbiome plays a role in metabolizing bile acids, which can affect cholesterol levels and cardiovascular health.

For the **endocrine system**, the microbiome plays a role in the metabolism and regulation of hormones. For instance, certain gut bacteria are involved in the metabolism of estrogens, which is vital for reproductive health.

Fifty-five-year-old Mary, struggling with menopausal symptoms and recurrent urinary tract infections, sought relief from a naturopathic doctor after traditional medications fell short. The doctor recommended a diverse probiotic and prebiotic regimen with strains specifically beneficial for the endocrine and urogenital systems. Within weeks, Mary experienced fewer hot flashes and mood swings, indicating improved hormone regulation. Furthermore, she saw significant improvements in her urogenital health, including a reduction in urinary tract infections. Motivated by these promising results, Mary integrated further lifestyle changes, promoting her gut health. Consequently, she experienced fewer menopausal symptoms, emotional balance, and overall enhanced quality of life, underscoring the power of targeted probiotics and gut-supporting lifestyle modifications.

In a rigorous 2020 study published in the Journal of Clinical Endocrinology & Metabolism, researchers evaluated the impact of Lactobacillus rhamnosus GG supplementation on glucose metabolism and inflammation in women with **Polycystic Ovary Syndrome (PCOS)**. The randomized, double-blind, placebo-controlled trial revealed that this probiotic significantly enhanced insulin sensitivity and curtailed systemic inflammation, offering a promising avenue for PCOS management.

An abundance of evidence and anecdotal reports suggest that adopting a diet rich in prebiotic fibers, probiotics, fermented foods, and diverse plant-based foods can significantly improve mood and cognitive function. Specific probiotics, known as psychobiotics, have been demonstrated in alleviating **depression and anxiety** symptoms by supporting the Hypothalamus-Pituitary-Adrenal (HPA) axis, **adrenal function**, and producing the calming neurotransmitter GABA.

Probiotic strains produce butyrate that mitigates anxiety and depression, as highlighted in a 2016 study in Gut Pathogens. Moreover, other strains have been shown to be highly effective in combating **mood disorders**, reducing **stress levels**, and enhancing **mental well-being**.

This is not just theoretical; a groundbreaking 2015 study published in Brain, Behavior, and Immunity involving forty participants established the remarkable benefits of Lactobacillus helveticus and Bifidobacterium longum in improving mental health. Those who took the probiotics experienced significant reductions in psychological distress, including depression, anger, and anxiety. This demonstrates the transformative potential of targeted probiotics, especially when combined, in fostering a strong gut-brain connection, alleviating stress, regulating cortisol, and enhancing mood and alertness.

The microbiome plays a crucial role in maintaining the body's systems and acts as a protector against chronic and autoimmune diseases while positively influencing various aspects of our health. Its vast size and diversity underscore its immense impact on our overall well-being.

As we now understand, the microbiome's influence extends far beyond digestive health, permeating every aspect of our being. Its impact on our overall health is profound, yet often underappreciated and misunderstood. Microbiome therapy and strategy hold a pivotal role, as they influence many systems including the cardiovascular, endocrine, skin, brain, immune and others; they are instrumental in the management of conditions such as Type 2 diabetes, chronic fatigue, celiac, and other autoimmune illnesses.

Moving forward, recognizing and maintaining a balanced microbiome will be instrumental in promoting optimal well-being and preventing a range of ailments. Continued exploration and appreciation of the microbiome's significance hold promise for advancements in medicine and personalized approaches to healthcare in the future. Embracing the consumption of probiotics as an enduring lifestyle choice is vital, as opposed to a temporary measure, thereby ensuring the continuous nurturing of this delicate internal garden for optimal health.

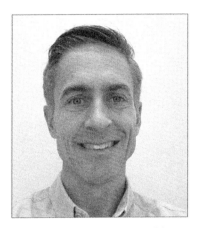

With a rich background in wellness, nutrition, and personalized functional medicine, **Mike** brings a combined experience of twenty years in the nutraceutical industry and nine years of assisting practitioners with complex cases, including those involving chronic illnesses and autoimmune disorders. Mike studied at Weber State University where he obtained a Bachelor's degree in Functional Nutrition, providing him with a solid foundation in understanding the pivotal role of how to personalize diet and nutrition in promoting health and managing diseases.

Mike further honed his expertise in this field by pursuing a Master's degree in Nutritional Sciences from the University of Utah. This advanced study expanded his understanding of human nutritional needs, metabolic pathways, and the connection between how diet and holistic health can help to overcome chronic illnesses.

Mike's work throughout these years has centered on the principle of optimizing patient outcomes. He is deeply committed to exploring and applying natural therapies and nutritional approaches that promote wellbeing, prevent illnesses, and aid in the management of health conditions. Mike strongly believes in the power of personalized functional medicine—an approach that treats the individual, not just the disease, and which has the potential to revolutionize healthcare as we know it. His ultimate goal is to create an overwhelmingly positive impact in the lives of clinicians, thereby transforming their businesses and empowering them to help their patients achieve healthier, more vibrant futures.

Made in the USA
Monee, IL
25 September 2023

43408736R00148